OPPOSING VIEWPOINTS® SERIES

I0811310

Genetic Engineering and Gene Therapy

Other Books of Related Interest

Opposing Viewpoints Series

Corporate Farming
DNA Testing and Privacy
Genetically Modified Foods and the Global Food Supply
Pesticides and GMOs

At Issue Series

Reproductive Rights
The Role of Science in Public Policy
Universal Health Care
Vaccination

Current Controversies Series

Attacks on Science
Genetic Engineering
The Industrial Food Complex
Medical Use of Illicit Drugs

> "Congress shall make no law … abridging the freedom of speech, or of the press."
>
> *First Amendment to the US Constitution*

The basic foundation of our democracy is the First Amendment guarantee of freedom of expression. The Opposing Viewpoints series is dedicated to the concept of this basic freedom and the idea that it is more important to practice it than to enshrine it.

OPPOSING VIEWPOINTS® SERIES

Genetic Engineering and Gene Therapy

Avery Elizabeth Hurt, Book Editor

GREENHAVEN PUBLISHING

Published in 2023 by Greenhaven Publishing, LLC
29 E. 21st Street
New York, NY 10010

First Edition

Cover image: Gorodenkoff/Shutterstock.com

Library of Congress Cataloging-in-Publication Data

Names: Hurt, Avery Elizabeth, editor.
Title: Genetic engineering and gene therapy / Avery Elizabeth Hurt, book editor.
Description: First edition. | New York : Greenhaven Publishing, 2023. | Series: Opposing viewpoints | Includes bibliographical references and index. | Contents: Genetic engineering and gene therapy. | Audience: Ages 15+ | Audience: Grades 10–12 | Summary: "Anthology of essays examining the issues of genetic engineering and gene therapy from technological, moral, and societal perspectives"— Provided by publisher.
Identifiers: LCCN 2021059184 | ISBN 9781534508712 (library binding) | ISBN 9781534508705 (paperback)
Subjects: LCSH: Gene therapy—Juvenile literature. | Genetic engineering—Juvenile literature.
Classification: LCC RB155.8 .G47 2023 | DDC 615.8/95—dc23/eng/20211208
LC record available at https://lccn.loc.gov/2021059184

Manufactured in the United States of America

Website: http://greenhavenpublishing.com

Contents

The Importance of Opposing Viewpoints 11
Introduction 14

Chapter 1: Should Gene Therapy Be Used to Cure Diseases?

Chapter Preface 18

1. Ethical Concerns of Gene Editing Must Be Discussed and Debated 19
   National Human Genome Research Institute
2. Some Gene Therapy Trials Offer False Hope 24
   Antonio Regalado
3. Gene Editing Technology Raises Ethical Questions That Go Beyond Medicine 31
   Raghav Ahooja
4. Using Gene Editing to Enhance Intelligence Is a Step Too Far 36
   Cary Funk and Meg Hefferon
5. We Need Guidelines in Place Now to Deal with the Potential Problems of Gene Editing Technology 44
   Tina Hesman Saey

Periodical and Internet Sources Bibliography 49

Chapter 2: Is It Ethical to Genetically Modify Animals for the Purpose of Scientific Research?

Chapter Preface 52

1. China Races Ahead with Genetic Engineering Research 53
   Jon Cohen
2. CRISPR Research Is Cruel to Animals 62
   Cruelty Free International
3. Americans Widely Support Genetic Engineering That Benefits Human Health but Not Other Uses 67
   Cary Funk and Meg Hefferon

4. Genome Editing Might Improve Animal Welfare, but It's Not That Simple **74**
Anna Wilkinson
5. The Ethics of Genetically Modifying Farm Animals Is Still a Work in Progress **81**
YourGenome
Periodical and Internet Sources Bibliography **86**

Chapter 3: Should We Genetically Modify Animals to Replace Extinct Animals?

Chapter Preface **88**
1. Genetic Engineering Could Save Our Planet's Biodiversity **89**
Andrew Moore
2. We Can't Bring Back Extinct Species (But We Might Get a Suitable Replacement) **95**
Chris Fitch
3. De-Extinction Is Too Risky **107**
David L. Strayer
4. Genetic Rescue Could Provide a Crucial Stop-Gap for Threatened Species **114**
Laura Poppick
5. Gene Drives Can Eliminate Invasive Species, but Researchers Must Proceed with Caution **122**
Kathiann Kowalski
Periodical and Internet Sources Bibliography **128**

Chapter 4: Should Genetically Modified Foods Be a Part of Our Food System?

Chapter Preface **131**
1. According to the FDA, Our Foods, GMO and Otherwise, Are Safe **132**
USFDA

2. GMO Salmon Is Only Safe If It Doesn't Get Out **138**
Jessie Rack

3. Gene Modification of Crops Can Reduce Hunger Around the Globe **143**
Utibe Effiong and Ramadhani Noor

4. CRISPR-Modified Crops Don't Count as GMOs **149**
Yi Li

5. We Should Genetically Disenhance Animals Used in Factory Farms **155**
Jonathan Latimer

Periodical and Internet Sources Bibliography **162**

For Further Discussion **164**

Organizations to Contact **166**

Bibliography of Books **170**

Index **172**

The Importance of Opposing Viewpoints

Perhaps every generation experiences a period in time in which the populace seems especially polarized, starkly divided on the important issues of the day and gravitating toward the far ends of the political spectrum and away from a consensus-facilitating middle ground. The world that today's students are growing up in and that they will soon enter into as active and engaged citizens is deeply fragmented in just this way. Issues relating to terrorism, immigration, women's rights, minority rights, race relations, health care, taxation, wealth and poverty, the environment, policing, military intervention, the proper role of government—in some ways, perennial issues that are freshly and uniquely urgent and vital with each new generation—are currently roiling the world.

If we are to foster a knowledgeable, responsible, active, and engaged citizenry among today's youth, we must provide them with the intellectual, interpretive, and critical-thinking tools and experience necessary to make sense of the world around them and of the all-important debates and arguments that inform it. After all, the outcome of these debates will in large measure determine the future course, prospects, and outcomes of the world and its peoples, particularly its youth. If they are to become successful members of society and productive and informed citizens, students need to learn how to evaluate the strengths and weaknesses of someone else's arguments, how to sift fact from opinion and fallacy, and how to test the relative merits and validity of their own opinions against the known facts and the best possible available information. The landmark series Opposing Viewpoints has been providing students with just such critical-thinking skills and exposure to the debates surrounding society's most urgent contemporary issues for many years, and it continues to serve this essential role with undiminished commitment, care, and rigor.

The key to the series's success in achieving its goal of sharpening students' critical-thinking and analytic skills resides in its title—

Opposing Viewpoints. In every intriguing, compelling, and engaging volume of this series, readers are presented with the widest possible spectrum of distinct viewpoints, expert opinions, and informed argumentation and commentary, supplied by some of today's leading academics, thinkers, analysts, politicians, policy makers, economists, activists, change agents, and advocates. Every opinion and argument anthologized here is presented objectively and accorded respect. There is no editorializing in any introductory text or in the arrangement and order of the pieces. No piece is included as a "straw man," an easy ideological target for cheap point-scoring. As wide and inclusive a range of viewpoints as possible is offered, with no privileging of one particular political ideology or cultural perspective over another. It is left to each individual reader to evaluate the relative merits of each argument—as he or she sees it, and with the use of ever-growing critical-thinking skills—and grapple with his or her own assumptions, beliefs, and perspectives to determine how convincing or successful any given argument is and how the reader's own stance on the issue may be modified or altered in response to it.

This process is facilitated and supported by volume, chapter, and selection introductions that provide readers with the essential context they need to begin engaging with the spotlighted issues, with the debates surrounding them, and with their own perhaps shifting or nascent opinions on them. In addition, guided reading and discussion questions encourage readers to determine the authors' point of view and purpose, interrogate and analyze the various arguments and their rhetoric and structure, evaluate the arguments' strengths and weaknesses, test their claims against available facts and evidence, judge the validity of the reasoning, and bring into clearer, sharper focus the reader's own beliefs and conclusions and how they may differ from or align with those in the collection or those of their classmates.

Research has shown that reading comprehension skills improve dramatically when students are provided with compelling, intriguing, and relevant "discussable" texts. The subject matter of these collections could not be more compelling, intriguing, or urgently relevant to today's students and the world they are poised to inherit. The anthologized articles and the reading and discussion questions that are included with them also provide the basis for stimulating, lively, and passionate classroom debates. Students who are compelled to anticipate objections to their own argument and identify the flaws in those of an opponent read more carefully, think more critically, and steep themselves in relevant context, facts, and information more thoroughly. In short, using discussable text of the kind provided by every single volume in the Opposing Viewpoints series encourages close reading, facilitates reading comprehension, fosters research, strengthens critical thinking, and greatly enlivens and energizes classroom discussion and participation. The entire learning process is deepened, extended, and strengthened.

For all of these reasons, Opposing Viewpoints continues to be exactly the right resource at exactly the right time—when we most need to provide readers with the critical-thinking tools and skills that will not only serve them well in school but also in their careers and their daily lives as decision-making family members, community members, and citizens. This series encourages respectful engagement with and analysis of opposing viewpoints and fosters a resulting increase in the strength and rigor of one's own opinions and stances. As such, it helps make readers "future ready," and that readiness will pay rich dividends for the readers themselves, for the citizenry, for our society, and for the world at large.

Introduction

> *"Americans have mixed views over whether the use of gene editing to reduce a baby's risk of serious disease that could occur over their lifetime is appropriate (60%) or is taking medical technology too far (38%)."*
>
> *—Pew Research Center*

Charles Darwin spent most of his life working out the theory of evolution by natural selection. He knew that traits, such as coat color, height, and so on, were passed down from parent to offspring. He explained how small changes, called mutations, could make an individual different from its parents and alter the course of a species. But he never understood exactly how those traits were passed from parent to offspring. In 1859, the year that Darwin published *On the Origin of Species*, no one else did either.

Swiss biochemist Johann Friedrich Miescher discovered DNA in 1869, but he didn't realize what he'd found. He called it "nuclein." Then in 1881, Albrecht Kossel, a German biochemist, figured out what "nuclein" was made of and gave it the name deoxyribonucleic acid (DNA). It was, he realized, the carrier of genetic information, the mechanism for heredity. But still it wasn't clear exactly *how* DNA worked that magic.

Other scientists discovered bits and pieces of the story, but it wasn't until the middle of the 20th century, more than 70 years after Darwin's death, that a team of researchers in England discovered the structure of DNA. Things went fast after that, very fast, because once scientists understood how DNA was put together, they were able to set about taking it apart.

By the late 20th century, scientists had discovered a group of DNA sequences in bacteria. These would soon be known as CRISPR. (CRISPR is an acronym for "clustered regularly interspaced short palindromic repeats." Now you see why everyone just calls it CRISPR, pronounced "crisper.")

By using an enzyme called Cas9 (CRISPR-associated protein 9), scientists can cut and splice the DNA of an organism. The technique is called CRISPR-Cas9. And it's difficult to overstate the importance of this discovery. Basically it's a tool that enables scientists to reprogram the cells of any organism.

The potential benefits are staggering. So are the potential pitfalls. Using CRISPR, we soon may be able to cure cancers, prevent genetic diseases such as sickle cell disease, create crops that can withstand climate change, make food more nutritious, and maybe even bring back extinct species. Scientists have been able to alter the genes of mice to prevent Duchenne muscular dystrophy, a devasting genetic disease. Researchers have created a mosquito that cannot transmit malaria, an infection that kills half a million people a year. And there is so much more that this technology can do, or will soon be able to do.

But the technology may have opened a Pandora's box. Once these altered organisms have been set loose in nature—including in the human genome—do we have any idea what will happen? Will we have any control over them?

Unintended consequences are not the only outcome to be feared. Should terrorists or lunatics use the technology to, say, alter a mosquito so that it transmitted a deadly and incurable disease, hundreds of millions of people could die. And CRISPR is remarkably easy to use. The risk is so great that the US director of national intelligence classified CRISPR a potential weapon of mass destruction.

Can we trust even scientists to use this technology responsibly? One of the no-go zones was thought to be altering the germline of humans—that is, making changes to the genome that could be passed down to children. However, in 2018, a Chinese scientist announced that he had successfully edited the DNA of human embryos, making the children-to-be less likely to get HIV, the virus that causes AIDS. The benefits weren't clear (the children were not at high risk of HIV to begin with), and the risks were, and still are, largely unknown. The scientific community was shocked and called for a moratorium on gene editing in embryos and germline cells. In 2020, the Chinese government sentenced the researcher to three years in prison for "illegal medical practice." But the genie is out of the bottle. What one rogue researcher can do, another can, too. The lesson learned here is that CRISPR is a remarkably inexpensive and easy technology to use, and it takes only a few irresponsible people crossing the line into the unknown to potentially create a nightmare of global proportions.

These questions and many more are on the minds of the authors of the viewpoints in *Opposing Viewpoints: Genetic Engineering and Gene Therapy*. In chapters titled "Should Gene Therapy Be Used to Cure Diseases?" "Is It Ethical to Genetically Modify Animals for the Purpose of Scientific Research?" "Should We Genetically Modify Animals to Replace Extinct Animals?" and "Should Genetically Modified Foods Be a Part of Our Food System?" viewpoint authors explore the latest controversies in the field of genetics. The questions are complex with no easy answers, but the viewpoints presented in this volume provide a variety of interesting and thoughtful approaches.

OPPOSING VIEWPOINTS® SERIES

Chapter 1

Should Gene Therapy Be Used to Cure Diseases?

Chapter Preface

Not too long ago, the notion of being able to cure diseases by tinkering with the genetic code was science fiction and only science fiction. Today it is very nearly reality. But all those science fiction stories may have helped prepare us for the many ethical challenges we would face once the technology was available. And that time is now. These are ethical challenges we are just beginning to have to confront.

Those challenges aren't just a matter of the risk-benefit equation of the new therapies. They involve everything from religious questions (are humans *meant* to interfere with the code of life?) to social questions (will this be a technology only for the wealthy?). And the social questions become even more difficult once gene therapy moves beyond the obvious benefits of curing cancer and preventing genetic diseases to the murkier ethics of changing genetic characteristics such as intelligence and athleticism in children before they are born—what one author calls "customizing" embryos.

The viewpoint authors in this chapter debate the use of gene therapy in curing diseases and also examine many of the complex and challenging questions that are being posed, or soon will be, about this revolutionary new technology. What shall we do with it? What should we absolutely never do with it? How should we regulate it? How can we keep unethical people from abusing the technology? And what are the consequences when this technology is not handled in a careful, appropriate way?

VIEWPOINT 1

> *"Most stakeholders agree that it is important to have continuing public deliberation and debate to allow the public to decide whether or not germline editing should be permissible."*

Ethical Concerns of Gene Editing Must Be Discussed and Debated

National Human Genome Research Institute

In the following viewpoint, the National Human Genome Research Institute begins by acknowledging the importance of public deliberation and debate about the issues surrounding gene editing technology. The viewpoint goes on to discuss specific ethical concerns, such as safety, justice, and equity. The National Human Genome Research Institute is an institute of the National Institutes of Health (NIH), the US government agency responsible for biomedical and public health research.

As you read, consider the following questions:

1. How has CRISPR technology changed the game when it comes to genome editing?
2. What, according to this viewpoint, is the difference between the terms *genome editing* and *gene editing*?
3. What are the issues of justice and equality brought up by this technology?

"What Are the Ethical Concerns of Genome Editing?" National Human Genome Research Institute.

The debate about genome editing is not a new one but has regained attention following the discovery that CRISPR has the potential to make such editing more accurate and even "easy" in comparison to older technologies.

Bioethicists and researchers generally believe that human genome editing for reproductive purposes should not be attempted at this time, but that studies that would make gene therapy safe and effective should continue.[1, 2] Most stakeholders agree that it is important to have continuing public deliberation and debate to allow the public to decide whether or not germline editing should be permissible. As of 2014, there were about 40 countries that discouraged or banned research on germline editing, including 15 nations in Western Europe, because of ethical and safety concerns.[3] There is also an international effort led by the US, UK, and China to harmonize regulation of the application of genome editing technologies. This effort officially launched in December 2015 with the International Summit on Human Gene Editing in Washington, DC.

NHGRI uses the term "genome editing" to describe techniques used to modify DNA in the genome. Other groups also use the term "gene editing." In general, these terms are used interchangeably.

Ethical Considerations

Safety

Due to the possibility of off-target effects (edits in the wrong place) and mosaicism (when some cells carry the edit but others do not), safety is of primary concern. Researchers and ethicists who have written and spoken about genome editing, such as those present at the International Summit on Human Gene Editing, generally agree that until germline genome editing is deemed safe through research, it should not be used for clinical reproductive purposes; the risk cannot be justified by the potential benefit. Some researchers argue that there may never be a time when genome editing in embryos will offer a benefit greater than that of existing technologies, such as preimplantation genetic diagnosis (PGD) and in-vitro fertilization (IVF).[4]

However, scientists and bioethicists acknowledge that in some cases, germline editing can address needs not met by PGD. This includes when both prospective parents are homozygous for a disease-causing variant (they both have two copies of the variant, so all of their children would be expected to have the disease); cases of polygenic disorders, which are influenced by more than one gene; and for families who object to some elements of the PGD process.[5, 6]

Some researchers and bioethicists are concerned that any genome editing, even for therapeutic uses, will start us on a slippery slope to using it for non-therapeutic and enhancement purposes, which many view as controversial. Others argue that genome editing, once proved safe and effective, should be allowed to cure genetic disease (and indeed, that it is a moral imperative).[6] They believe that concerns about enhancement should be managed through policy and regulation.

Lastly, commenters on the issue are concerned that the use of genome editing for reproductive purposes will be regulated differently inside and outside of the US, leading to uses considered objectionable to the American public. These arguments cite the largely self-regulated environments of the reproductive clinics that offer PGD and IVF[7, 8] and the existing differences in regulations among different countries.[9]

Informed Consent

Some people worry that it is impossible to obtain informed consent for germline therapy because the patients affected by the edits are the embryo and future generations. The counterargument is that parents already make many decisions that affect their future children, including similarly complicated decisions such as PGD with IVF. Researchers and bioethicists also worry about the possibility of obtaining truly informed consent from prospective parents as long as the risks of germline therapy are unknown.[10]

Justice and Equity

As with many new technologies, there is concern that genome editing will only be accessible to the wealthy and will increase existing disparities in access to health care and other interventions. Some worry that taken to its extreme, germline editing could create classes of individuals defined by the quality of their engineered genome.

Genome-Editing Research Involving Embryos

Many people have moral and religious objections to the use of human embryos for research. Federal funds cannot be used for any research that creates or destroys embryos. In addition, NIH does not fund any use of gene editing in human embryos.

While NIH will not fund gene editing in human embryos at this time, many bioethical and research groups believe that research using gene editing in embryos is important for myriad reasons, including to address scientific questions about human biology, as long as it is not used for reproductive purposes at this time.[11, 12] Some countries have already allowed genome-editing research on nonviable embryos (those that could not result in a live birth), and others have approved genome-editing research studies with viable embryos.[13, 14] In general, research that is conducted in embryos could use viable or nonviable embryos leftover from IVF, or embryos created expressly for research. Each case has its own moral considerations.

References

1. National Academies of Sciences, E., Medicine. (2017). Human Genome Editing: Science, Ethics, and Governance. Washington, DC: The National Academies Press.

2. The Hinxton Group. (2015). Statement on Genome Editing Technologies and Human Germline Genetic Modification. Retrieved from http://www.hinxtongroup.org/Hinxton2015_Statement.pdf

3. Araki, M., & Ishii, T. (2014). International regulatory landscape and integration of corrective genome editing into in vitro

fertilization. Reprod Biol Endocrinol, 12, 108. doi:10.1186/1477-7827-12-108

4. Lanphier, E., Urnov, F., Haecker, S. E., Werner, M., & Smolenski, J. (2015). Don't edit the human germ line. Nature News, 519(7544), 410. doi:10.1038/519410a
5. Hampton, T. (2016). Ethical and Societal Questions Loom Large as Gene Editing Moves Closer to the Clinic. JAMA, 315(6), 546-548. doi:10.1001/jama.2015.19150
6. Savulescu, J., Pugh, J., Douglas, T., & Gyngell, C. (2015). The moral imperative to continue gene editing research on human embryos. Protein Cell, 6(7), 476-479. doi:10.1007/s13238-015-0184-y
7. Ishii, T. (2017). Germ line genome editing in clinics: the approaches, objectives and global society. Brief Funct Genomics, 16(1), 46-56. doi:10.1093/bfgp/elv053
8. Park, A. (2016). UK Approves First Studies Using New Gene Editing Technique. Time Health.
9. Araki, M., & Ishii, T. (2014). International regulatory landscape and integration of corrective genome editing into in vitro fertilization. Reprod Biol Endocrinol, 12, 108. doi:10.1186/1477-7827-12-108
10. Lanphier, E., Urnov, F., Haecker, S. E., Werner, M., & Smolenski, J. (2015). Don't edit the human germ line. Nature News, 519(7544), 410. doi:doi:10.1038/519410a
11. The Hinxton Group. (2015). Statement on Genome Editing Technologies and Human Germline Genetic Modification. Retrieved from http://www.hinxtongroup.org/Hinxton2015_Statement.pdf
12. National Academies of Sciences, E., Medicine. (2017). Human Genome Editing: Science, Ethics, and Governance. Washington, DC: The National Academies Press.
13. Callaway, E. (2016). UK scientists gain licence to edit genes in human embryos. Nature News, 530(7588), 18. doi:doi:10.1038/nature.2016.19270
14. Cyranoski, D., & Reardon, S. (2017). Chinese scientists genetically modify human embryos. Nature News. doi:doi:10.1038/nature.2015.17378

Viewpoint 2

> *"[Pay-to-play trials] are not necessarily unethical. But you should scrutinize why the patient is being asked to pay. If it's a valid trial, why isn't … there other funding?"*

Some Gene Therapy Trials Offer False Hope

Antonio Regalado

Experimental therapies, like gene therapies, raise many ethical questions. And not all of those questions have to do with the risks of the treatments. In the following viewpoint, Antonio Regalado explores gene therapy trials that are not funded by government or industry, but instead require patients (or in this case the patients' families) to pay for the treatment—what he calls "pay-to-play" trials. Especially in the case of very ill children, trials such as these could be giving parents false hope. Antonio Regalado is a senior editor at MIT Technology Review.

As you read, consider the following questions:

1. Why does the author write that, although "pay-to-play" trials are not illegal, their ethics may be borderline?
2. What are the realistic chances that these children will be cured?
3. What do the researchers in this story have at stake? What about the parents?

When Gary Landsman prays, he imagines he is in Israel and his sons Benny and Josh are running toward him. They are wearing yarmulkes, and the cotton fringes called tzizit fly out from their waistbands. He opens his arms ready for a tackle.

The reality is Benny and Josh both have Canavan disease, a fatal inherited brain disorder. They are buckled into wheelchairs, don't speak, and can't control their limbs.

On Thursday, April 8, in Dayton, Ohio, Landsman and his family rolled the older boy, Benny, into a hospital where over several hours, neurosurgeons drilled bore holes into his skull and injected trillions of viral particles carrying the correct version of a gene his body is missing.

The procedure marked the climax of a four-year quest by the Landsman family, who live in Brooklyn, New York, to obtain a gene therapy they believe is the only hope to save their kids.

MIT Technology Review first profiled the Landsmans' odyssey in the cover story of our 2018 special issue on precision medicine. Advances in gene therapy technology are making it possible to treat genetic diseases like hemophilia. But because Canavan is an ultra-rare disease, few companies are working on a cure. So the family financed the daring gene treatment on their own, using funds they raised online.

Impressive advances in genome sequencing, gene replacement, and gene editing mean, in theory, thousands of rare genetic diseases could be treated. But because companies aren't leading the way, parents say, they are being forced to embark on multimillion-dollar quests to finance the needed experiments. Adding to the ethical dilemma: in some cases, parents are designating their own children as the first recipients.

The trial in Dayton, for instance, is prioritizing children whose families have been able to raise funds to underwrite the experiment, whose costs so far are close to $6 million. "It raises the eternal equity question of who gets access to trials and who doesn't," says Alison Bateman-House, a bioethicist at New York University who is studying ethical issues in pediatric gene-therapy trials.

The Landsman family has raised more than $2 million, and families from Russia, Poland, Slovakia, and Italy have also used cash donations to secure spots in the trial. A Russian family even posted a copy of an invoice for "gene-therapy treatment" in the amount of $1,140,000, which included $800,000 to offset costs of manufacturing the genetic treatment being used in the trial.

According to the Russian family's urgent fundraising appeal, if they failed to pay that amount, their toddler Olga "will not receive the only chance for recovery—an expensive treatment in the United States." They ended up contributing at least $700,000.

While such "pay-to-play" trials are legal, they do raise red flags, including questions about whether parents—and financial

First Human CRISPR Gene Therapy Trials Show Promise

Until February of this year, when pharmaceutical companies CRISPR Therapeutics and Vertex began a large global trial into a treatment called CTX001, no human outside of China had been officially treated with a CRISPR-based gene editing therapy.

CTX001 was developed to treat two types of inherited blood disease, beta-thalassemia and sickle cell disease. Both conditions are caused by a mutation in a single gene and the treatment involves engineering a patient's stem cells with a single genetic change designed to raise levels of fetal hemoglobin in red blood cells.

The newly announced data from the first two patients treated with CTX001 is nothing short of extraordinary. The first patient was treated with the CRISPR therapy at the beginning of 2019 for transfusion-dependent beta-thalassemia. The patient's illness was so severe they required around 16 blood transfusions every year. Nine months after the single CTX001 treatment the patient was completely independent of the need for blood transfusions and their total hemoglobin levels were near normal.

The second patient, treated for sickle cell disease, demonstrated similar remarkable responses to the one-off gene therapy treatment. Four months after the CTX001 infusion the patient's total hemoglobin donors—understand that most experimental treatments fail. "They are not necessarily unethical. But you should scrutinize why the patient is being asked to pay," says Bateman-House. "If it's a valid trial, why isn't the NIH [National Institutes of Health] interested, or a biotech company? Why isn't there other funding?"

Will It Work?

Canavan disease is caused when a child inherits two broken copies of a gene called *ASPA*. Without the enzyme that *ASPA* produces, the brain can't correctly form the nerve bundles that transmit signals in the brain. The result, for Benny and Josh, is that the boys can't speak or control their limbs, and their cognition is limited.

> levels had returned to normal and many of the disease symptoms had disappeared.
>
> Both patients did suffer from a small number of serious adverse events following the CTX001 treatment, However, the researchers conducting the trial are confident none of these side effects were related to the gene therapy. Instead, these side effects seem primarily related to a pre-CTX001 treatment involving the elimination of pre-existing mutated bone marrow cells to enable the healthy CRISPR-edited cells to reproduce.
>
> Still, these initial results are as positive as one could hope for at this stage, establishing CRISPR gene editing as having exciting curative potential in human subjects. Whether the treatment holds for extended periods of time and demonstrates longer safety profiles is yet to be determined. But, these early results are leaving researchers cautiously optimistic.
>
> "The data we announced today are remarkable and demonstrate that CTX001 has the potential to be a curative CRISPR/Cas9-based gene-editing therapy for people with sickle cell disease and beta thalassemia," says CEO of Vertex, Jeffrey Leiden. "While the data are exciting, we are still in the early phase of this clinical program."
>
> **"Encouraging Early Results from First Human CRISPR Gene Therapy Trials," by Rich Haridy, New Atlas, November 19, 2019.**

"They are like infants in ALS bodies," says Paola Leone, the researcher at Rowan University in New Jersey who conceived the gene therapy and led the effort to get a clinical trial started.

The trial in Dayton seeks to use viruses to deliver working copies of the *ASPA* gene to kids' brain tissue. That's what occurred Thursday at the Dayton Children's Hospital. After Benny was greeted by a golden retriever who cheers patients up, brain surgeons drilled into his skull and then used a needle to introduce 40 trillion virus particles.

Leone's scientific bet is that adding correct copies of *ASPA* to specific brain cells called oligodendrocytes could stop the disease from progressing, and maybe allow for some recovery. The treatment has been effective in mice, she says, but "is that going to work in patients? The only way is to test it."

Parents as Scientists

There are by now a half-dozen examples of gene-therapy treatments funded by families aiming to treat their own kids, and more such experiments are planned. Scientists have even begun developing hyper-personalized medicine tailored to individual children who suffer from unique genetic problems.

These desperate efforts ask parents to overcome nearly impossible obstacles. They must become experts in drug development, raise millions, and tirelessly cajole scientists. Few people can pull it off.

"There are a lot of people who know how to do gene therapy, but the knowledge is all fragmented, and so much can go wrong," says Sanath Kumar Ramesh, a software developer whose son is afflicted by a different rare disease. Ramesh founded an organization, Open Treatments, that is building software families can use to organize gene-therapy research, including steps such as hiring scientists to create animal models of an illness.

"I think in the future, the distinction between scientists and parents is going to be blurred," he says.

For parents whose kids have already been accepted into the Dayton trial, gene therapy may be their last chance. One of them is Meagan Rockwell, a nail technician in Cedar Rapids, Iowa, whose daughter, Tobin Grace, now three and half, was diagnosed with Canavan in 2018.

"They told us sorry, there is nothing we can do—no treatment, no cure—you will be lucky if she sees her fifth birthday. It was a hard blow, to know your only child has a life-limiting brain disease," Rockwell says.

Rockwell says she found out about Leone's gene-therapy effort online and eventually raised more than $250,000. "At the time, Tobin was the youngest person in the US with Canavan, and I think that played a huge factor in her acceptance," she says, adding that Leone tells parents money puts them at the front of the line but doesn't guarantee treatment.

Bateman-House, the bioethicist, says another risk is whether parents can really judge the benefits of an experimental procedure in a "dispassionate" way, especially if they have sunk a fortune into the effort. "It's not only that their child is facing a dangerous condition; it's that their blood, sweat, and tears is what is funding this intervention," she says. "It could be incredibly difficult for a parent to change their mind and say 'We are not going to do this.'"

Hope Versus Risk

The Dayton study currently has enough supplies of the genetic drug to treat only nine or 10 children. It was manufactured in Spain, but only after the researchers and families overcame what they call an ordeal of red tape, delays, and obstacles, some thrown up by government regulators who decide which genetic treatments can be tried and whether trials are properly planned.

At one point, in 2019, the Landsmans took their sons to the US Food and Drug Administration for a meeting they landed after dozens of calls to lawmakers. "Beforehand we were a case number in their big pile of paper," says Jennie Landsman, the boys' mother. "They had very technical objections. In the meeting we held up Benny and Josh, and we said 'We hope this issue that is so technical isn't going to stop the treatment.'"

The Dayton trial won a greenlight in December and began barely in time for Benny, who will hit the age cutoff of five years in June. "Benny is the pilot. Benny is the 'God, we hope this works' kid," says Rockwell, who doesn't yet have a date for her daughter's procedure.

What's the chance the therapy works? Gene-replacement techniques have been having notable successes, curing kids who don't have immune systems, and preventing brain diseases. Since 2017, a small number of gene therapies have also been approved for sale in the US, at prices as high as $2.1 million per child.

Record prices have stoked interest among specialist biotech companies, which now see a business even in super-rare diseases. One, called Aspa Therapeutics, says it has plans to initiate a different Canavan gene-therapy trial. Its CEO, Eric David, estimates there are 1,000 children alive with the disease in the US and Europe. "That, for us, is enough," he says.

There's no certainty gene therapy will succeed in Canavan. Even if the corrected gene stops the disease from progressing, the kids' brains may have already been irreversibly damaged.

"I hope she will sit up on her own, maybe say Mommy and Daddy," says Rockwell of her daughter. "I am hopeful, but it is purely experimental. We are handing our babies over to science and hoping and praying it works." It will be a month before doctors know if the new gene is functioning in Benny's brain, but likely much longer to know of any effect on his symptoms.

In a message to donors, Gary Landsman addressed what he called the "loaded" question of what he expects the procedure to achieve.

"I've pondered this question over and over and over again," he wrote. "Is it OK to want more? Is it OK to want to hold their hands as they walk beside me? Is it OK to want to hear them speak to me? Perhaps I am playing a dangerous game with my psyche. But I think the hope it provides is worth the risk."

Viewpoint 3

> *"Do we fast forward using techno solutionism or do we let evolution do its thing? Where do we draw the line?"*

Gene Editing Technology Raises Ethical Questions That Go Beyond Medicine

Raghav Ahooja

Treating serious illnesses is not gene therapy's only potential use. The ethical dilemmas presented by using gene therapy to genetically enhance children make the dilemmas of treatment seem mild. In the following viewpoint, Raghav Ahooja considers the ethical issues posed when technology enables people to genetically "customize" their children before birth. At the time of this writing, Raghav Ahooja was a law student at Rajiv Gandhi National University of Law, Punjab focusing on tech law and policy and constitutional law.

As you read, consider the following questions:

1. How could changing a baby's genes permanently change the lineage of the family?
2. According to the author, how do Germany's laws differ from those in the US in this regard?
3. Why would a blanket ban on genetic editing violate human dignity, according to the author's interpretation of German law?

"Gene Editing: Do We Have the Right to Genetically Enhance Our Children?" by Raghav Ahooja, The Leaflet, September 19, 2020. Reprinted by permission.

We are at crossroads wherein we may be able to customize and design the futures of our future generations. Lawmakers, thus, need to solve the ethical dilemmas brought about by such giant scientific leaps.

Even though it may sound like science fiction, the future is here.

Gene editing for therapeutic purposes (namely gene therapy) is being conducted for the removal of diseases in humans and foetuses both. When changes are made to the somatic cells, the modifications aren't hereditary. However, when the changes are made to the sperm, egg, or embryo, the modifications are transferred on to the next generation. It is done through a process called "germline" gene editing.

It seems like German philosopher Neitzsche's post-human concept of Übermensch (translated as beyond-man or superman) might become real. Using a technology known as CRISPR, one can not only treat diseases but also customize a baby in terms of intelligence, athleticism, and so on. This can permanently enhance the lineage of the family.

Law and Gene Editing

Somatic gene editing has been approved in countries like the United States, although with restrictions. It is for the Courts and lawmakers to decide whether this right to "enhance" children for their own welfare falls within the right to privacy of the parents, or whether the state has a right to curtail such an action.

According to American jurisprudence, there is a private realm of family life that the state cannot enter. Yet time and again the state has entered this realm, claiming a legitimate interest in regulating the family, especially for the welfare of the child. Thus, whilst there exists a right to privacy under the Fourteenth Amendment, it is not absolute.

In the famous case of *Roe v. Wade*, the United States Supreme Court held that the right to abortion is embedded in the right to privacy of the parent bearing the child. While the judgment was pro-choice, gene editing doesn't quite fit the bifurcated and antagonistic pro-choice v. pro-life debate. It gives parents the choice to genetically edit their children, and the aim of such editing inter alia is to eradicate disease and enhance children for their own welfare.

Germany, as opposed to the US, recognises the unborn as an individual with a "genetically determined" identity, which is unique and inseparable. According to German courts, as the unborn baby grows, it does not only develop into a human being but develops as a human being and is worthy of human dignity. Such human dignity would also include the right to live a dignified life, which is free of disease. Therefore, a blanket ban on gene editing would be violative of human dignity.

It is quite clear that therapeutic gene editing is not violative of human dignity, insofar its aim is to eradicate disease. However, such human dignity also includes the right to free development of personality.

A plain reading of the German constitutional text would suggest that non-therapeutic editing for personality factors is violative of human dignity. But to the contrary, heritable gene editing for purposes such as personality building will be permissible for strengthening the autonomy of the child. Furthermore, it must be for the welfare of the child and must not restrict the free development of their personality. A thumb rule could be—whether the child would subsequently consent to such a modification.

In India, guidelines permitting development of therapeutic gene editing products were introduced. Currently, heritable gene editing can only be done for purposes of experimentation and the embryo cannot have a life beyond 14 days. Thus, heritable gene editing is yet not fully permitted in India. However, there is scope as the Indian Supreme Court in K.S. Puttaswamy (2017) recognised that the right to privacy encompasses family affairs and childrearing. This would possibly entail the parents' right to enhance their child as an extension of their right to choose.

Child, State and Parents in Gene Editing

It is an established position in law that technology mustn't be prohibited due to a mere possibility of harm. Rather, a positivist approach must be adopted so as to do the greatest good to the greatest number. In fact, a recent report by a German government-appointed council of experts stated that heritable gene editing is not violative of human dignity.

Further, a joint statement by the councils of the United Kingdom, France, and Germany stated that heritable gene editing is permissible. However, there must be a risk assessment and the risk must be brought down to a minimum acceptable level.

The question, when looked at more deeply, is whether the personality and well-being of future generations ought to be subjected to medical decisions or not.

Thus, there is a tripartite relationship of the right of the parents to choose the genetic make–up of their children, the right of the state to regulate such an act, and the right of the unborn baby to consent to such editing.

The American Supreme Court in *Planned Parenthood v. Casey* has reiterated that the matters involving the intimate choices of a person are central to dignity and autonomy protected under "liberty" enshrined in the American Constitution. And that at the heart of this liberty lies the right to define one's own concept of existence, of meaning, of the universe, and of the mystery of human life, without the interference of the state.

Where Does That Leave Us?

Ultra-modern technologies such as artificial wombs make one think whether a birth is really an event, or a "process," and if so then where does the "process" begin?

Partial ectogenesis (the growth of a baby outside the womb) is already happening. But in time, we might be able to carry out full ectogenesis. As the reliability of such technologies increases, so does their capability. The potential to live outside the mother's womb as opposed to the usual 24 weeks would begin right from the stage of development of the foetus, which is at 8 weeks. Further, with the help of biotech, the ability of an unborn baby to live outside the mother's womb might begin right at fertilisation.

The American Courts have held that an individual whether single or married has the right to privacy which the state cannot infringe. Thus, even a single parent, out of wedlock, can bear such a child and the right to genetically edit unborn babies would be extended to them. The mother and father would be on an equal footing while deciding whether to genetically edit the baby or not.

The aim of the process of childrearing is to produce children with favourable traits and personality and allow them to have a dignified life.

In the first such successfully germline edited babies, scientists predict that it might have actually led to having enhanced their ability to learn and form memories. In another case of successful gene therapy, young children were saved from potentially deadly diseases and lives of isolation.

Therefore, the moot question is: Do we fast forward using techno solutionism or do we let evolution do its thing? Where do we draw the line? Should one circumscribe the limits of technology, or let it take a well-designed course?

Believe it or not, the future is here.

Where does that leave us?

It is for us to decide.

Viewpoint 4

> *"Those most familiar with gene editing are more likely than those with no familiarity to also anticipate downsides."*

Using Gene Editing to Enhance Intelligence Is a Step Too Far

Cary Funk and Meg Hefferon

In the following viewpoint, researchers at Pew Research examine the data on Americans' views about editing the genes of unborn children. Not surprisingly, most Americans support the idea of using gene editing technology to prevent or cure illness. An almost equal number think using it to boost a baby's intelligence is going too far. However, the answers vary depending on the exact question and the demographic of the people answering. Cary Funk is director of science and society research, and Meg Hefferon is a research analyst at the Pew Research Center.

As you read, consider the following questions:

1. Based on the surveys cited, have Americans' views on this issue changed?
2. How do women's views differ from men's views on this issue?
3. How do religious people's views differ?

"Public Views of Gene Editing for Babies Depend on How It Would Be Used," by Cary Funk and Meg Hefferon, Pew Research Center, July 26, 2018.

Americans' views on the appropriateness of changing a baby's genetic characteristics depend in large part on the intended purpose and on whether or not human embryos would be used in testing these techniques. A majority of Americans support the idea of using gene editing with the goal of delivering direct health benefits for babies, but at the same time, a majority considers the use of such techniques to boost a baby's intelligence something that takes technology "too far."

About seven-in-ten Americans (72%) say that changing an unborn baby's genetic characteristics to treat a serious disease or condition that the baby would have at birth is an appropriate use of medical technology, while 27% say this would be taking technology too far. A somewhat smaller share of Americans say gene editing to reduce a baby's risk of developing a serious disease or condition over their lifetime is appropriate (60% say this, while 38% say it would be taking medical technology too far). But just 19% of Americans say it would be appropriate to use gene editing to make a baby more intelligent; eight-in-ten (80%) say this would be taking medical technology too far.

These are some of the findings from a new Pew Research Center survey conducted April 23-May 6, 2018, among 2,537 U.S. adults.

While public discussions about potentially altering a baby's genetic makeup have been ongoing for decades, the development of a new gene-splicing technology—known as CRISPR—has accelerated the debate and brought new urgency to better understanding public opinion about gene editing as well as the broader social, ethical and policy implications ahead.

Previous Pew Research Center surveys have tracked public opinion about gene editing using different question wording and, in some cases, different polling methodologies. As such, those findings are not directly comparable to this new survey. However, the broad pattern—that public support for gene editing varies with its intended purpose—is consistent with a 2016 study that explored public views about the possibility of using gene editing to "enhance" a baby's health over the course of their lifetime and a 2014 survey.

Regardless of the intended purpose of gene editing, experts acknowledge that further development of these techniques will likely involve testing in human embryos. In August 2017, research scientists in the United States reported the first successful use of gene editing in human embryos to eliminate an inherited condition. When asked to consider the possibility that the development of gene editing would involve testing on human embryos, one-third of Americans (33%) say this would be appropriate while about two-thirds (65%) say this would be taking medical technology too far.

The 2016 Pew Research Center survey using different question wording found that most adults said testing on human embryos to develop gene editing would make gene editing less acceptable for them.

Public Views of Gene Editing Vary by Religious Commitment, Gender, Levels of Science Knowledge and Familiarity with Gene Editing

Several patterns emerge in public opinion about gene editing in these varying contexts. There are large differences in acceptance of gene editing between the highly religious and less religious. In addition, there is a gender gap in views about gene editing, with women less accepting of it than men. People with higher levels of science knowledge and greater familiarity with gene editing also tend to be more accepting of it.

Religious Americans Are More Likely to View Gene Editing Negatively

Americans who are high in religious commitment—that is, those who attend religious services at least weekly, pray at least daily and say that religion is very important in their lives—are less inclined than those with either medium or low levels of religious commitment to say that gene editing is an appropriate use of medical technology. For example, those high in religious commitment are closely divided over whether it is appropriate to use gene editing to reduce a baby's risk of disease later in life; 46% say this is appropriate, while 53% consider it taking technology too far. In contrast, roughly three-quarters of those low in religious commitment (73%) say gene editing to reduce a baby's risk of developing a serious disease or condition is an appropriate use of medical technology. And, while a 57% majority of those high in religious commitment say gene editing to treat a congenital disorder in a baby is an appropriate use of medical technology, a much larger share of those with low religious commitment (82%) say this is appropriate.

Those with high levels of religiosity also stand out when considering the possibility that development of gene editing would entail testing on human embryos. An overwhelming majority of those high in religious commitment (87%) say this would be taking medical technology too far; just 11% of this group says this would be appropriate. In contrast, 55% of those low in religious commitment say that development of gene editing techniques that require testing on human embryos would be an appropriate use of medical technology.

The differences by religiosity in views on the appropriateness of gene editing tend to persist even when statistically controlling for other factors such as gender, race and ethnicity, age, and education that are related to religious beliefs and practices.

There are also differences in views about gene editing by religious affiliation, particularly if such techniques would involve embryonic testing. Just 11% of white evangelical Protestants say that if development of gene editing techniques required testing on human embryos, it would be an appropriate use of medical technology.

By contrast, about half of the religiously unaffiliated (52%), including 79% of atheists and 57% of agnostics, say that embryonic testing to develop gene editing techniques would be an appropriate use of medical technology.

Men Are More Accepting Than Women of Using Gene Editing to Change a Baby's Genetic Makeup

Men are more inclined than women to view gene editing as an appropriate use of medical technology, regardless of its intent. About two-thirds of men (65%) believe that gene editing to reduce a baby's risk of developing a serious disease later in life is an appropriate use of medical technology, compared with 54% of women. And men (76%) are more supportive than women (68%) of using gene editing to treat a congenital disorder.

Similarly, more men (43%) than women (24%) are accepting of gene editing technology if it required embryonic testing to develop.

Women tend to have higher levels of religious commitment, on average, but differences by gender tend to hold even when controlling for religiosity and other factors in statistical models.

Previous Pew Research Center surveys in 2016 and 2014, while not directly comparable due to different polling methods and question wording, have also found that women tend to be less accepting than men when it comes to gene editing for babies.

Americans with High Levels of Science Knowledge Are More Likely to View Gene Editing in a Positive Light

People high in science knowledge—based on a nine-item index—tend to be more accepting of using gene editing for babies. Some 86% of those with high science knowledge believe it is appropriate to use gene editing to treat a congenital disorder, compared with 58% of those with low science knowledge. And, 71% of those with high science knowledge say it is appropriate to use gene editing to reduce a baby's risk of disease that would occur later in life, compared with 49% of those with low science knowledge.

However, few Americans say it is appropriate to use gene editing to make a baby more intelligent, regardless of their level of science knowledge.

Judgments on the appropriateness of gene editing also follow a similar pattern by education level, which is closely linked with science knowledge. Those with a postgraduate degree are more accepting of gene editing for treating or reducing the risk of a disease than those with a high school degree or less.

Americans Who Report Familiarity with Gene Editing Are More Inclined to See It as Appropriate

People who say they have heard at least a little about gene editing that can be used to change a baby's genetic characteristics are more likely than those who have heard nothing at all to say gene editing would be appropriate in each of the circumstances considered in this survey.

A Pew Research Center survey in 2016 found a similar tendency for those who report familiarity with gene editing to express more interest in and acceptance of using these technologies to enhance a baby's health over the course of their lifetime.

Americans Are More Likely to Anticipate Negative Than Positive Effects from Gene Editing

Although gene editing for babies is still in development, a separate April 2018 survey found that about half of Americans (52%) believe it is likely that within the next 50 years, we will be able to eliminate almost all birth defects by manipulating the genes of an embryo before a baby is born. In the current survey, as people think about a future with possible widespread use of gene editing to change a baby's genetic makeup, more anticipate negative than positive effects on society.

Specifically, a majority of Americans (58%) believe gene editing will very likely lead to increased inequality because it will only be available to the wealthy. Some 54% of Americans anticipate a slippery slope, saying it's very likely that "even if gene editing is used appropriately in some cases, others will use these techniques in ways that are morally unacceptable." And, 46% expect it is very likely that gene editing techniques will be used before we fully understand how they affect people's health.

Far smaller shares see positive outcomes as very likely if gene editing for babies were to become widely available. Roughly two-in-ten Americans (18%) say it is very likely that development of these techniques will pave the way for new medical advances that benefit society as a whole. Another 42% say this is fairly likely to occur, while 38% consider this not too or not at all likely. Just 16% see the widespread use of gene editing as very likely to help people live longer and better quality lives. About half (48%) say this is fairly likely, while 34% say this outcome is not too or not at all likely.

Women are more inclined than men to expect negative effects if gene editing becomes widely available, in keeping with gender differences over acceptance of gene editing. For example, larger shares of women than men say this technology will lead to an increase in inequality as it will only be available for the wealthy (63% say this is very likely vs. 52% of men) or say it will be used in morally unacceptable ways (57% vs. 51%). And although only minorities of men and women see positive effects as very likely, men are somewhat more inclined to anticipate positive outcomes.

Expectations also vary by self-reported familiarity with gene editing. Those who have heard a lot about gene editing to change a baby's genetic characteristics are more inclined to anticipate positive outcomes from its widespread use. Some 36% of this group thinks it is very likely that the widespread availability of gene editing would pave the way for new medical advances that are beneficial to society, compared with about half as many of those who have heard a little or nothing about gene editing (16%).

However, those most familiar with gene editing are more likely than those with no familiarity to also anticipate downsides. About two-thirds of those who have heard a lot about gene editing (64%) say it is very likely that widespread availability of gene editing will increase inequality because the technology will primarily be available only for the wealthy, compared with 53% of those who have heard nothing about using gene editing to change a baby's genetic characteristics. And, 65% of those who have heard a lot about gene editing think it's very likely that others will use these techniques in morally unacceptable ways, while 54% of those who have heard a little and 52% of those who have heard nothing about gene editing say this.

A similar pattern occurs with levels of science knowledge. A larger share of people with high science knowledge anticipate positive outcomes from the widespread availability of gene editing than those with low science knowledge. At the same time, those with high science knowledge are at least equally likely as those with low science knowledge to think negative effects from the widespread availability of gene editing are very likely.

The American public also tends to be skeptical about whether medical experts fully comprehend the health consequences of gene editing. A 36% minority of Americans believe that medical researchers understand the health effects of gene editing for babies either very (7%) or fairly well (29%), while 62% say medical researchers do not understand the health effects at all or not too well.

Familiarity with gene editing is linked with beliefs about medical researchers' understanding of it. About half of those who have heard a lot about gene editing for babies (51%) say that medical researchers understand the health effects of gene editing for babies at least fairly well, compared with three-in-ten of those who have heard nothing at all (30%). However, level of science knowledge based on a nine-item index is not related to views on this issue; 36% of those with high science knowledge and 40% of those with low science knowledge believe that medical researchers understand the health effects of changing a baby's genetic characteristics at least fairly well.

There are no or only modest differences on this question by gender or religious commitment.

Viewpoint 5

"An organization similar to the World Anti-Doping Agency, which oversees use of performance-enhancing drugs in sports, might be set up to keep an eye out for unauthorized gene editing."

We Need Guidelines in Place Now to Deal with the Potential Problems of Gene Editing Technology

Tina Hesman Saey

One of the more vexing questions about gene editing concerns the potential to make alterations to heritable traits, those traits that are transmissable from parents to their offspring. In the following viewpoint, Tina Hesman Saey explores a report by the International Commission on the Clinical Use of Human Germline Genome Editing that offers guidelines for making such changes in the event that society eventually deems the gene-editing of babies to be acceptable. Tina Hesman Saey is a reporter covering molecular biology for Science News.

"Strict New Guidelines Lay Out a Path to Heritable Human Gene Editing," by Tina Hesman Saey, Society for Science & the Public, September 3, 2020. Reprinted by permission.

As you read, consider the following questions:

1. What prompted the formation of the International Commission on the Clinical Use of Human Germline Genome Editing?
2. Why do some critics say it is too early for these guidelines?
3. What might rogue scientists do with this technology, according to sources cited in this article?

Gene editing to make heritable changes in human DNA isn't yet safe and effective enough to make gene-edited babies, an international scientific commission says. But in a Sept. 3 report, the group laid out a road map for rolling out heritable gene editing should society decide that kind of DNA alteration is acceptable.

The International Commission on the Clinical Use of Human Germline Genome Editing formed after a Chinese scientist announced in 2018 that he had created two gene-edited baby girls, sparking outrage (SN: 11/27/18). In its first official weigh-in on the issue, the group lays out strict scientific criteria that would need to be met before heritable gene editing could be tried clinically. If countries can't ensure that all of those criteria are met, heritable gene editing shouldn't be approved, the commissioners say.

Still, some critics charge that even presenting such criteria is premature. The science should wait until society decides whether to allow gene editing that can affect future generations, they say.

Gene editing involves changing a single DNA letter, or base, in a gene. Many different technologies, including CRISPR/Cas9, base editors (SN: 3/5/19) and engineered proteins called zinc finger nucleases and TALENs (SN: 11/6/15), can be used to make edits at precise locations in DNA. Although accuracy of editing has improved, there are still concerns that gene editors will make unwanted, "off-target" changes elsewhere in DNA that might cause harm. Technologies to ensure every cell in an embryo contains the desired change—and only that change—also still need work, the commission says.

"It's accurate and efficient enough to do in animals," but editing in human embryos requires much more precision, Haoyi Wang, a geneticist and molecular and stem cell biologist at the Chinese Academy of Sciences' Institute of Zoology in Beijing said September 3 during a webinar to discuss the report.

Scientists are already testing CRISPR gene editing to correct the inherited blood disorders sickle-cell anemia and beta-thalassemia and an inherited form of blindness called Leber congenital amaurosis 10 in adults (SN: 8/14/19). Those edits are in adult cells and can't be carried into future generations.

But altering DNA in the human germ line—embryos, eggs, sperm or the cells that give rise to them—would create changes that could be passed on to future generations. Many people, including scientists, are concerned that rogue scientists wouldn't stop at editing out diseases and would create "designer babies" with enhanced athletic ability, intelligence or other desirable traits.

The commission proposes that human germline editing should be restricted to serious genetic diseases caused by specific versions of single genes that are virtually guaranteed to cause the disease if inherited. Such disorders include Duchenne muscular dystrophy, Tay-Sachs disease and cystic fibrosis. Children who inherit these disorders die young or have serious medical problems.

The commission also specified that before human germline editing is considered, no other way of ensuring a couple can produce embryos without the disease-causing genetic variants should be available. That essentially winnows the eligible list down to couples in which both parents have two copies of recessive disease-causing variants, or couples in which one parent has two copies of mutations that cause a dominant genetic disorder, such as Huntington's disease, which results from inheriting a single copy of a faulty gene.

Perhaps 20 families around the world would meet these strict criteria, Michèle Ramsay, a human geneticist at the University of the Witwatersrand in Johannesburg, said September 3 during a news briefing.

So the commission also decided that some families with less serious disorders, but who have little chance of producing embryos without the disease-causing variants, would also be eligible. One example is familial hypercholesterolemia, an inherited form of high cholesterol that leads to early heart disease and death. That and other disorders are carried by a high proportion of people in parts of the world where marriage between cousins is common. Gene editing might be an option when 25 percent or fewer of a couple's embryos would be free of the disease-causing mutation.

Even then, such couples must already have attempted in vitro fertilization with a technique called preimplantation genetic testing to screen out embryos that carry the faulty version of the gene. "We're not thinking there are going to be a lot of people" that are qualified to take part in the initial research, Ramsay said. "There are no floodgates that are going to be opened." If the technology is both safe and effective in those few families, it might then be considered for other conditions.

The commission recommends more research on using stem cells to produce eggs and sperm in lab dishes, which could then be used to create embryos that don't carry genetic diseases. Such research has been done in mice (SN: 5/18/17), but is in its infancy with human cells, said Richard Lifton, a human geneticist at the Rockefeller University in New York City.

Heading off hubris was one of the commission's main concerns, Lifton said. The report also recommends establishing an international scientific advisory board to evaluate the state of the technology and consult on applications to do such heritable or germline editing.

An organization similar to the World Anti-Doping Agency, which oversees use of performance-enhancing drugs in sports, might be set up to keep an eye out for unauthorized gene editing, Lifton suggested. Reining in rogue scientists would also require setting up a way for whistleblowers to report possible unapproved research.

The report is "appropriately cautious and thoughtful and written with a clear appreciation for what's been going on in the world," said Kyle Orwig, an infertility researcher at the University of Pittsburgh who was not involved with the commission. "It's a bit aspirational because it raises questions about whether individual countries are willing to submit to international oversight," he added.

What's more, setting up global governance to prevent scientists from going rogue may not be as effective as laying out a clear moratorium or ban, says Katie Hasson, program director for genetic justice at the nonprofit Center for Genetics and Society, based in Berkeley, Calif.

Whether to allow changes to DNA that can be inherited by future generations is a decision that affects the whole human species, and should be an international consensus rather than a single country's decision, Wang said.

This report handled only the scientific aspects of gene editing. An upcoming report from the World Health Organization will tackle ethical and societal issues surrounding gene editing.

Hashing out how to do germline editing before society has indicated its desire to do so is backward, Hasson says. "The question has been and still is whether we want to move forward with editing the genes and traits of future generations," she says. "To skip ahead to how . . . seems like getting ahead of things a bit."

There is still a need for broad societal conversations about the technology. More than 70 countries already have laws that prohibit germline editing, and a moratorium and other laws might effectively stop the technology from moving forward, Hasson says. "There's no reason this should be inevitable. Laying out this path in advance makes it seem more inevitable and pushes us toward that conclusion."

Periodical and Internet Sources Bibliography

The following articles have been selected to supplement the diverse views presented in this chapter.

Bhaargavi Ashok and Jack Karsten, "Is There a Responsible Way Forward for Gene Editing?" Brookings, October 29, 2019, https://www.brookings.edu/blog/techtank/2019/10/29/is-there-a-responsible-way-forward-for-gene-editing/.

Jon Cohen, "Did CRISPR Help—or Harm—the First-Ever Gene-Edited Babies," *Science*, August 1, 2019, https://www.science.org/content/article/did-crispr-help-or-harm-first-ever-gene-edited-babies.

Graham Duggan, "The Future Is Here: Three Ways Gene Editing Could Change the World," The Nature of things, CBC, https://www.cbc.ca/natureofthings/features/the-future-is-here-three-ways-gene-editing-could-change-the-world/.

Katie Hafner, "Once Science Fiction, Gene Editing Is Now a Looming Reality," *New York Times,* July 22, 2020, https://www.nytimes.com/2020/07/22/style/crispr-gene-editing-ethics.html.

Elizabeth Kolbert, "CRISPR and the Slice to Survive," *New Yorker*, January 11, 2021, https://www.newyorker.com/magazine/2021/01/18/crispr-and-the-splice-to-survive.

Joe Ruff, "Catholic Ethics and Gene Editing," *Catholic Spirit*, April 8, 2019, https://thecatholicspirit.com/news/local-news/catholic-ethics-and-gene-editing/.

Tina Rulli, "Using CRISPR to Edit Eggs, Sperm or Embryos Does Not Save Lives," Stat, October 15, 2019, https://www.statnews.com/2019/10/15/reproductive-crispr-does-not-save-lives/.

Mark Shwartz, "Target, Delete, Repair: CRISPR Is a Revolutionary Gene-Editing Tool, but It's Not Without Risk," *Stanford Medicine,* Winter 2018, https://stanmed.stanford.edu/2018winter/CRISPR-for-gene-editing-is-revolutionary-but-it-comes-with-risks.html.

Kyle Smith, "The Gene Revolution Is Already Here," *National Review*, March 13, 2020, https://www.nationalreview.com/2020/03/documentary-human-nature-explores-genetics-revolution/.

Rob Stein, "He Inherited a Devastating Disease. A CRISPR Gene-Editing Breakthrough Stopped It," NPR, June 26, 2021, https://www.npr.org/sections/health-shots/2021/06/26/1009817539/he-inherited-a-devastating-disease-a-crispr-gene-editing-breakthrough-stopped-it.

World Health Organization, "Human Genome Editing: A Framework for Governance," July 12, 2021, https://www.who.int/publications/i/item/9789240030060.

Sarah Eekhoff Zylstra, "Christians to Science: Leave Our Bodies How God Made Them," *Christianity Today*, July 26, 2016, https://www.christianitytoday.com/news/2016/july/christians-science-leave-bodies-alone-pew-human-enhancement.html.

OPPOSING VIEWPOINTS® SERIES

CHAPTER 2

Is It Ethical to Genetically Modify Animals for the Purpose of Scientific Research?

Chapter Preface

In the previous chapter, viewpoint authors considered the question of whether gene editing technology should be used to treat illness. But before genetic engineering can be used as therapy for human illnesses, the technology has to be developed and tested. This typically involves using the techniques on animals. And that raises a slew of issues. Is this just one more way that animals can be mistreated in science labs? Do the potential benefits justify the possible cruelty? Or is there an actual net gain for animals since the technology can possibly be used to make their lives easier?

On top of that, CRISPR-Cas9 has upped the game for researchers working in this field. Because it's remarkably easy to make these changes in animals, some argue that researchers may be tempted to tinker and tweak in ways that are not necessary or even truly beneficial for anyone, animal or human.

Others point out that humans have been changing the genomes of animals ever since the beginning of agriculture (and in ways that benefit humans and often make animals even more miserable). It's just that until recently, we've done it the old-fashioned way, using the slow process of selective breeding. Now, with CRISPR, we can do it in a flash.

One argument against the speedy method of genetic tinkering is the potential for unintended consequences. Some critics point out that we don't know the long-term results of a given genetic change. For example, altering mosquitoes so that they cannot breed could save hundreds of thousands of humans from dying of malaria. But do we understand the insect's role in its complex ecosystem well enough to make that change?

The viewpoint authors in this chapter grapple with these issues and more, including a deep dive into US public opinion about genetic engineering on animals.

Viewpoint 1

> *"It just takes time for people to catch up and move into the preclinical models and then get enough evidence because no one wants to be the first there and have it turned into a disaster."*

China Races Ahead with Genetic Engineering Research

Jon Cohen

In the following viewpoint, Jon Cohen discusses Chinese research using CRISPR technology on monkeys, dogs, rats, mice, and rabbits to develop animal models of human diseases such as muscular dystrophy, autism, and cancer. In addition, genetic engineering is being used to develop organs for transplant. China has a robust scientific culture, and its government is pouring lots of money into this research. This may put China ahead of other countries that are taking a slower approach to the technology. Jon Cohen is a staff writer for Science.

"China's CRISPR Push in Animals Promises Better Meat, Novel Therapies, and Pig Organs for People," by Jon Cohen, American Association for the Advancement of Science, July 31, 2019. Reprinted by permission.

As you read, consider the following questions:

1. According to the viewpoint, why is China ahead of the West in animal research on genetic engineering?
2. Why are the Chinese editing the genomes of so many different animals?
3. What uses might these animals have besides medical treatments in humans?

Early one February morning, researchers harvest six eggs from a female rhesus macaque—one of 4000 monkeys chirping and clucking in a massive outdoor complex of metal cages here at the Yunnan Key Laboratory of Primate Biomedical Research. On today's agenda at the busy facility, outside Kunming in southwest China: making monkey embryos with a gene mutated so that when the animals are born 5 months later, they will age unusually fast. The researchers first move the eggs to a laboratory bathed in red light to protect the fragile cells. Using high-powered microscopes, they examine the freshly gathered eggs and prepare to inject a single rhesus sperm into each one. If all goes well, the team will introduce the genome editor CRISPR before the resulting embryo begins to grow—early enough for the mutation for aging to show up in all cells of any offspring.

But as often happens when eggs are retrieved, all does not go well. Only one egg in this morning's batch is mature enough to fertilize. "We were a little unlucky today," says Niu Yuyu, who with facility director Ji Weizhi runs the gene-editing research. The group can afford a little bad luck, though. Through a combination of patience, ingenuity, and enormous animal resources, the team has already used CRISPR to create an astonishing range of genome-edited monkeys to serve as models for studying human diseases.

Ji, Niu, and colleagues were the first to harness CRISPR in monkeys, as they reported in 2014, and they remain leaders in the field. They've built on that success, exploiting CRISPR's speed and precision to create monkey models of muscular dystrophy, autism, and cancer. In a tie with developmental biologist Yang Hui and co-workers at Shanghai's Institute of Neuroscience (a branch of the Chinese Academy of Sciences, CAS), they were first to use CRISPR in monkeys to introduce, or knock in, a gene—a particularly difficult feat that the two teams reported in back-to-back papers in 2018 in *Cell Research*.

The team also collaborated with He Jiankui, well before the Chinese biophysicist created the first CRISPR-edited human babies. Almost 2 years ago, in a proof of principle for He's infamous experiment, they knocked out in monkey embryos the gene for the immune cell protein CCR5, a mutation that makes humans resistant to infection with the most commonly transmitted variant of HIV. That work leaves them uneasy today. "We had no idea he was going to do this in a human being," Niu says, stressing that their study had yet to evaluate how the editing affected the monkeys when news of the edited babies broke. "It's unbelievable."

China now has at least four groups of CRISPR researchers doing gene editing with large colonies of monkeys. "The most startling part of what is coming out of China is seeing how they have just a brute-force approach," says reproductive biologist Jon Hennebold at the Oregon National Primate Research Center in Hillsboro. "The level of animal support they have to do those experiments is really astounding."

It's not just monkeys. China's researchers have racked up a long list of CRISPR firsts in dogs, mice, rats, pigs, and rabbits. That research promises higher quality meats, disease-resistant livestock, and new medical treatments and organs for human transplantation. So far, many of the animals are simply proofs of concept. Despite the multitude of CRISPR-altered monkeys, for example, Chinese teams have published "very little follow-up in terms of characterizing what these mutations mean from a [disease] model or a treatment perspective," Hennebold says.

But few people doubt that China will persist with its animal-editing binge. "This is a country and a culture that really values science and technology," says Jennifer Doudna of the University of

California, Berkeley, who helped develop CRISPR into an editing tool. "Their government has put very serious money into it, and they're walking the walk."

To get a feel for one of China's advantages, ask Hennebold—one of the few U.S. researchers using CRISPR to develop monkey models of disease—how many edited monkey embryos he has transferred. "You're going to laugh," he says. "Maybe 10." In contrast, Ji and Niu routinely implant embryos with the same CRISPR edit into 50 to 100 surrogate females. Another group—also at the Institute of Neuroscience—recently combined cloning and CRISPR to create 325 monkey embryos with the same mutation, one that disrupts circadian rhythms in people and is connected to sleep disorders, diabetes, and cancers. After implanting the embryos into 65 surrogate females, the team produced five genetically identical monkeys with the disorder.

In addition to having access to large colonies of monkeys and other species, animal researchers in China face less public scrutiny than counterparts in the United States and Europe. Ji, who says his primate facility follows international ethical standards for animal care and use, notes that the Chinese public has long supported monkey research to help human health. "Our religion or our culture is different from that of the Western world," he says. Yet he also recognizes that opinions in China are evolving. Before long, he says, "We'll have the same situation as the Western world, and people will start to argue about why we're using a monkey to do an experiment because the monkey is too smart, like human beings."

And then there's money: massive—if hard to quantify—government investment in both new facilities and ambitious research projects. As a result, China has become the center of the CRISPR animal kingdom, attracting top researchers. "In the States, it is harder to do monkey studies, so I moved back," says Yang, who did a postdoc in the United States and now is part of China's Thousand Talents Program, which aims to reverse the brain drain.

One major Chinese effort to edit animals traces its origins to 1998, when developmental biologist Lai Liangxue left China to join a lab at the University of Missouri in Columbia run by Randall Prather, a reproductive physiologist studying pigs. Prather, Lai, and co-workers set out to genetically engineer a pig whose organs could be transplanted into humans without rejection. Human immune systems won't tolerate cross-species, or "xeno," transplants because many pig genes code for incompatible proteins, and the Prather group wanted to cripple production of one protein that triggers particularly strong antibody responses. Four years later, the team reported in *Science* that it had engineered the world's first knockout pig.

"It took us so much time and so much money," Lai says, because the team had to rely on an imprecise and inefficient combination of transgenic and cloning technologies. The cumbersome knockout process required inserting a bacterial gene that would land randomly in the genome, which risked accidentally turning on a cancer gene or causing other problems. Over the next 10 years, Lai says, the team and others created only a few more genetically modified pigs.

In 2007, Lai returned to China and set up labs in Guangzhou and at Jilin University in the northeastern city of Changchun. By 2013, when other groups first showed CRISPR could alter animals, his team had adopted earlier genome-editing tools dubbed zinc fingers and transcription activatorlike effector nuclease (TALEN). With zinc fingers, Lai's team could edit a pig embryo in 2 to 3 months, and TALEN dropped the timeline to a month. "But with CRISPR, in just 1 week you can get everything done," Lai says. Everyone in his lab—nearly 30 people—began to use CRISPR to edit rabbits, dogs, and pigs.

To date, they have successfully made 40 different genetic modifications in pigs with CRISPR. "He's doing great stuff," Prather says. "I've trained all my competition over there, and I've trained them well."

Over the past decade, most of Lai's work has focused on creating pig models of human disease, ultimately to test new medicines. At his pig facility near Jiangmen, about a 2-hour drive from his lab, dozens of swine with edited genomes fill three barns. Lai has engineered some to age prematurely or develop neurodegenerative afflictions that mimic diseases such as Alzheimer's, Parkinson's, amyotrophic lateral sclerosis (Lou Gehrig's disease), and Huntington. Lai's group has also used CRISPR to knock in a humanized gene for albumin, a blood product given in cases of traumatic shock or liver failure. Lai hopes the protein, purified from the blood of the pigs, will enter human trials next year.

Across the country at CAS's Institute of Zoology in Beijing, geneticist Zhao Jianguo—another Prather alumnus—uses CRISPR to engineer improved pigs for the pork industry. He and colleagues 2 years ago endowed their pigs with a gene for uncoupling protein 1, which is found in most mammals and helps them form heat-producing brown fat. Swine, however, have lost the protein, and newborn pigs often die from hypothermia. Pigs with the gene restored by CRISPR stay warmer in cold environments, Zhao's group reported in 2017. The pigs also have about 5% less white fat, which makes for leaner meat. Colleagues on the same campus, led by Wang Haoyi and Zhou Qi, used CRISPR to make a genetic change that speeds growth in pigs, meaning farms could produce meat faster.

The Chinese groups and others are also turning to CRISPR to thwart several diseases that often devastate the pig industry. A gene added with CRISPR made pigs resistant to classical swine fever, Lai reported late last year, together with Ouyang Hongsheng and colleagues at Jilin University. Months earlier, Prather's team had reported creating pigs altered to resist the industry's costliest infection, porcine reproductive and respiratory syndrome virus.

When those advances will reach farmers in China is not clear, Zhao says. "The big barrier for Chinese companies is they don't want to put too much money into genetic modification for pig breeding because right now we don't have a timeline about how long it will take to get the genetically altered pig into the market," he says. China has not yet decided whether or how it will regulate

CRISPR-modified food, casting a pall of uncertainty over the efforts. "It is moving, but the progress is very slow."

Both the U.S. Food and Drug Administration (FDA) and China's Ministry of Agriculture now regulate CRISPR-modified pigs like old-school genetically modified organisms, which are severely restricted in both countries. That "just doesn't make sense to me," Prather says, who notes that the genetic changes introduced by CRISPR are often indistinguishable from natural mutations. Genus, a U.K.-based company, is counting on China to reconsider its current policy. Genus licensed the technology to commercialize Prather's virus-protected pigs and in May formed a collaboration with a Chinese company to bring them to market there—a process the firm says could take several years.

When Lai returned to China, he wanted to continue the xenotransplantation work he had begun in Prather's lab but couldn't get funding. "The Chinese government was not interested," he says. But over the past few years, attitudes have shifted. The government now strongly backs efforts by Lai and others to create pig organs that could help people with eye problems, diabetes, kidney and liver failure, and heart disease.

China has a critical organ shortage—300,000 people in need and 10,000 organs available—transplant specialist Deng Shaoping of Sichuan Provincial People's Hospital in Chengdu and his co-authors explained in February in a review article in *Xenotransplantation*. The shortage, they say, was exacerbated by the government's 2015 decision to stop harvesting organs from executed criminals. Now, they wrote, "China has the potential to become a world-renowned pig organ center, with the perspective of minimizing or even eliminating the current organ shortage for transplantation."

International science teams are joining the effort, with some starting commercial ventures in China. One such company is Qihan Biotech in Hangzhou, which collaborates with eGenesis of Cambridge—both co-founded by Harvard University's George Church, a CRISPR pioneer, and Yang Luhan, who earned her Ph.D.

in his lab. They are building on an advance the team reported 2 years ago, when they showed that CRISPR could remove dozens of genetic sequences called endogenous retroviruses from pigs.

Those vestiges of ancient infections theoretically could harm humans who receive pig organ transplants, although other researchers downplay the risk. "I don't think [the sequences are] a very big issue," Zhao says. "The really big barrier is the immunorejection, not the viruses." No one knows how many pig genes will ultimately have to be knocked out to prevent human rejection of their organs—estimates range as high as 20—but to date, Lai and co-workers have disabled four in one animal, and at least five other groups in China also are targeting such genes, according to the *Xenotransplantation* article.

As the final step before a human trial, researchers routinely put gene-edited pig tissue or organs into a monkey, widely considered the best testing ground for predicting human responses. Few Chinese investigators have made that crucial step. Lai's team hopes to transplant a CRISPR-modified pig organ to a monkey next year, which he notes will require a large, skilled team of surgeons and specialists. "It takes so many people to care for the animal, and it's very, very expensive."

Peter Cowan, a leading xenotransplantation researcher at St. Vincent's Hospital in Melbourne, Australia, says China's recent push to get back into the field, aided by CRISPR, puts them a bit behind the leading groups. "It just takes time for people to catch up and move into the preclinical models and then get enough evidence because no one wants to be the first there and have it turned into a disaster."

Competition is stiffening. A South Korean group hopes to transplant CRISPR-engineered pig corneas or insulin-making islet cells into people in clinical trials starting in May 2020. By the end of next year, a U.S. team led by Revivicor in Blacksburg, Virginia, that works with David Cooper of the University of Alabama in Birmingham may test a pig kidney with nine modified genes in people on dialysis. The team is already testing their kidneys in baboons but still needs FDA approval to conduct the human trial. "The timeline is very close now because we've got so much encouraging data," Cooper says.

Lai may be a bit behind in the xenotransplant race, but he's also competing on more fronts than almost any other CRISPR animal researcher. About 150 kilometers from where his pigs live, a research farm on the forested banks of the Lian'an reservoir houses 2000 beagles used in a variety of scientific experiments. The two most famous are Lai's creations: a female named Tiangou, the heavenly dog in Chinese legend that eats the sun or the moon, and Hercules, a male whose name more clearly reflects why they have received international attention.

Lai used CRISPR in the two dogs to cripple a gene that normally constrains muscle mass. The beagles are 5 years old now, and their jaws have a hint of pit bull. Their pectoral and thigh muscles bulge, resembling the sculpted humans who compete in bodybuilding contests. But the dogs are sweet, gentle beagles through and through. They hold the distinction of being the world's first, and to date only, dogs modified with CRISPR.

Although Lai acknowledges that breeders might want to engineer dogs that can jump higher and run faster, he created Tiangou and Hercules in 2015 simply to show that CRISPR works in canines and can be done safely. "This genotype is really easy to observe, so people at the regulatory agency can see it with their own eyes," Lai says.

The dogs may be just for show. But researchers in China and abroad say the country's industrial-scale effort to transform animals with CRISPR will soon yield real payoffs for fundamental research, agriculture, and medicine.

Lai, for one, says his university has just invested 60 million yuan (nearly $9 million) in a new, higher-tech facility for both his pig and rabbit research. "Come back next year," he says. "The whole thing will change."

Viewpoint 2

> *"In the UK alone, half of all experiments (around 2 million) carried out in 2017 involved the production and breeding of GM animals that were not used in further research."*

CRISPR Research Is Cruel to Animals

Cruelty Free International

In the following viewpoint, Cruelty Free International cites statistics showing how many animals are used in genetic engineering research and describes cruel experiments on animals. The authors argue that using CRISPR on animals is not only cruel but has little if any benefit to justify the suffering of the animals. Cruelty Free International is a UK-based organization that works to end experiments on animals worldwide.

As you read, consider the following questions:

1. Why is CRISPR research particularly hard on animals, according to the viewpoint?
2. Why does this author say that the claims that researchers have found a cure for Duchenne muscular dystrophy are exaggerated?
3. Why does the author argue that animals make poor models for studying disease in humans?

"A New Threat to Animals—the CRISPR GM Technique," Cruelty Free International, October 19, 2018. Reprinted by permission.

The use of genetically modified (GM) animals in science is a significant cause of the year-on-year increase in the number of animals used in experiments around the world.

For example, in the UK alone, half of all experiments (around 2 million) carried out in 2017 involved the production and breeding of GM animals that were not used in further research, and 38% of actual experiments used GM animals (Ref. 1). The welfare concerns for these animals are considerable, and suffering has been acknowledged at every step of the GM process (Ref. 2, 3).

A new method called the CRISPR/Cas9 system, or simply CRISPR, has entered the limelight mainly because, compared to other methods, it is an inexpensive, relatively simple and quick way of producing GM animals. It has also been claimed to not only be more accurate than traditional methods but to actually help reduce animal numbers (because it is so accurate that less animals might be wasted). Unfortunately, neither claim is true.

In fact, CRISPR is only likely to exacerbate the current ethical and welfare problems associated with the production of GM animals by simply increasing the number of GM animals created. This will more than offset any potential benefits that may arise from its possible greater efficiency in the future.

While CRISPR may be more efficient and specific at generating desired genetic modifications, there is evidence that it is far from good enough. Studies have shown that the efficiency of CRISPR to insert or "knock-in" a particular gene in an animal is less than 4% (Ref. 4) or less than 1% (Ref. 5), while the efficiency to delete or "knock-out" a gene is around 7% (Ref. 5). Furthermore, it appears that CRISPR introduces unwanted or "off-target" mutations (in addition to those that are intended). While the degree is open to question, these unintended genetic modifications can be numerous, and may well have serious consequences.

Perhaps even more troubling is the increasing use of CRISPR in larger animals. Some scientists are calling for more GM monkeys or dogs to be created, in an effort to "fix" rodent models of human diseases that are increasingly acknowledged as failures (Ref. 6, 7).

Just last month, two experiments that involved the use of CRISPR in monkeys and dogs were published in high-profile scientific journals *Nature* and *Science*:

- In a particularly cruel experiment on monkeys in China, researchers wanted to determine the function of a gene thought to play a significant role in ageing. This gene was "knocked-out" of GM monkeys using CRISPR. To generate these monkeys, 48 embryos were transferred into 12 surrogate mothers, and of these, only 4 were successfully impregnated, with 3 completing their pregnancy and giving birth. Sadly, all 3 babies died soon after birth, and showed "retarded development" that resembled that of a 2- to 4-month old foetus. Shockingly, the authors plan to continue to create these monkeys to study miscarriages and stillbirths (Ref. 8). We are writing to *Nature* to complain about their decision to publish this unethical study, which has little scientific merit.
- Scientists at the UK's Royal Veterinary College have been breeding dogs with Duchenne muscular dystrophy (DMD), a rare and devastating muscle-wasting disease, in a bid to find a cure for the condition in humans. According to a journalist who visited the breeding facility, dogs with the disease were visibly weak and were seen stumbling and struggling to walk (Ref. 9). The scientists claim that they have managed to "cure" DMD in dogs thanks to CRISPR, which they used to edit a mutated gene to once again produce dystrophin, an important muscle protein. Regardless of the hype, the study has already been widely criticised for several reasons, including its short duration (less than 2 months), the small number of dogs used (4 beagles), and uncertainty surrounding the long-term effects of CRISPR, e.g. possibility that cancer-causing mutations may be introduced. Further, while the dogs were able to produce dystrophin, there was little evidence they regained any muscle function. Sadly, the researchers plan to conduct longer lasting experiments on a larger number of dogs (Ref. 10).

Fortunately, there are scientists who do not support the breeding and use of GM dogs and monkeys, and who warn against it for both scientific (e.g. they are difficult to successfully create) and animal welfare reasons (Ref. 11).

Animals have always been bad models for humans due to species differences, and no amount of genetic modification can remedy that, even if those techniques were perfect. Instead of trying to "improve" GM processes, we should be working towards the greater adoption and use of technologically advanced and human-specific alternatives such as 3D culture of human stem cells, human organoids and tissue/body-on-a-chip technologies, which are already being used to investigate a wide range of diseases.

Next year the European Commission President's European Group on Ethics in Science and New Technologies (EGE) will be reviewing the ethics of gene editing techniques and will be discussing whether it is ethical to produce GM monkeys. We will be ensuring our concerns are shared with them.

References:

1. UK Home Office. (2018). Statistics of Scientific Procedures on Living Animals: Great Britain 2017. [online] Available at: https://www.gov.uk/government/statistics/statistics-of-scientific-procedures-on-living-animals-great-britain-2017.
2. LASA (Laboratory Animal Science Association). (2008). Position paper: transgenics. [online] Available: http://www.lasa.co.uk/PDF/position_transgenics.pdf.
3. BVAAWF/FRAME/RSPCA/UFAW Joint Working Group on Refinement. (2003). Refinement and reduction in the production of genetically modified mice. Laboratory Animals;37 Suppl 1:S1-S49.
4. Genome editing using CRISPR/Cas9-based knock-in approaches in zebrafish. (2017). Methods 121, 77-85.
5. Ultra-superovulation for the CRISPR-Cas9-mediated production of gene-knockout, single-amino-acid substituted, and floxed mice. (2016). Biology Open 5, 1142-1148.

6. Refining strategies to translate genome editing to the clinic. (2017). Nature Medicine 23, 415-423.
7. Opportunities and challenges in modeling human brain disorders in transgenic primates. (2016). Nature Neuroscience 19, 1123-1130.
8. SIRT6 deficiency results in developmental retardation in cynomolgus monkeys. (2018). Nature, 560: 661-665.
9. Beagles bred with muscular dystrophy offer "hope of a human cure." (2015). The Guardian, 14 November: http://www.theguardian.com/science/2015/nov/15/beagles-study-hope-cure-muscular-dystrophy.
10. In dogs, CRISPR fixes a muscular dystrophy. (2018). Science, 36(1): 835.
11. Every silver lining has a cloud: the scientific and animal welfare issues surrounding a new approach to the production of transgenic animals. (2014). Alternatives to Laboratory Animals 42, 137-145.

Viewpoint 3

> *"Emerging developments in animal biotechnology raise new social, ethical and policy issues for society, including the potential impact on animal welfare."*

Americans Widely Support Genetic Engineering That Benefits Human Health but Not Other Uses

Cary Funk and Meg Hefferon

In the following viewpoint, Cary Funk and Meg Hefferon present the results of a Pew Research Center survey on Americans' views on genetic engineering. The public's views vary quite a bit depending on what the technology is being used for and how great the benefits are likely to be. However, views also vary across demographics. The viewpoint also includes sample comments by the people surveyed. Cary Funk is director of science and society research, and Meg Hefferon is a research analyst at the Pew Research Center.

"Most Americans Accept Genetic Engineering of Animals That Benefits Human Health, but Many Oppose Other Uses," by Cary Funk and Meg Hefferon, Pew Research Center, August 16, 2018.

As you read, consider the following questions:

1. Why might Americans widely support genetically engineering mosquitoes to prevent them from reproducing but not support changing aquarium fish to make them glow?
2. What was the most common reason for opposing the genetic engineering of mosquitoes?
3. What different demographic groups are represented by these findings?

As Americans consider the possible uses of genetic engineering in animals, their reactions are neither uniformly accepting nor resistant; instead, public reactions vary depending on the mechanism and intended purpose of the technology, particularly the extent to which it would bring health benefits to humans.

Presented with five different scenarios of animal genetic engineering that are currently available, in development or considered possible in the future, Americans provide majority support only for the two that have clear potential to pre-empt or ameliorate human illness.

The survey's most widely accepted use of genetic intervention of animals involves mosquitoes. Seven-in-ten Americans (70%) believe that genetically engineering mosquitoes to prevent their reproduction and therefore the spread of some mosquito-borne diseases would be an appropriate use of technology, while about three-in-ten (29%) see the use of genetic engineering for this purpose as taking technology too far.

And a 57% majority considers it appropriate to genetically engineer animals to grow organs or tissues that could be used for humans needing a transplant.

But other uses of animal biotechnology are less acceptable to the public, including the creation of more nutritious meat for human consumption (43% say this is appropriate) or restoring an extinct animal species from a closely related species (32% say this is appropriate). And one application that is already commercially available is largely met with resistance: Just 21% of Americans consider it an appropriate use of technology to genetically engineer aquarium fish to glow using a fluorescence gene, while 77% say this is taking technology too far.

These are some of the findings from a new Pew Research Center survey, conducted April 23-May 6 among a nationally representative sample of 2,537 U.S. adults that looks at public views about genetic engineering of animals—a term that encompasses a range of biotechnologies that can add, delete or change an animal's existing genetic material and thereby introduce new traits or characteristics.

Although most Americans are largely in agreement that using genetic engineering in mosquitoes to prevent the spread of mosquito-borne illnesses is appropriate, views about other uses of genetic engineering of animals considered in the survey differ by gender, levels of science knowledge and religiosity. Men are more accepting of these uses of technology than women, those with high science knowledge are more accepting than those with medium or low science knowledge and those low in religious commitment are more accepting than those with medium or high levels of religious commitment.

For example, about two-thirds of men (65%) see genetic engineering of animals to grow human organs or tissues for transplants as appropriate, compared with about half of women (49%). Also, Americans with high science knowledge (72%) are more inclined than those with medium (55%) or low (47%) science knowledge to say this would be appropriate. And a larger share of those with low religious commitment (68%) than medium (54%) or high (48%) religious commitment consider genetic engineering of animals to grow human organs or tissues for transplants to be appropriate.

Emerging developments in animal biotechnology raise new social, ethical and policy issues for society, including the potential impact on animal welfare.

The survey finds that the 52% of Americans who in general oppose the use of animals in scientific research are, perhaps not surprisingly, also more inclined to consider specific uses of genetic engineering of animals to be taking technology too far.

There are large differences between these groups when it comes to using animal biotechnology for humans needing an organ or tissue transplant and the idea of using such technology to produce more nutritious meat.

Reasoning Behind Public Qualms over Animal Biotechnology

To better understand people's beliefs about genetic engineering of animals, the survey asked a subset of respondents to explain, in their own words, the main reason behind their view that genetic engineering in each of these circumstances would be taking technology too far.

A common refrain in these responses raised the possibility of unknown risks for animals, humans or the ecosystem. Some saw these technologies as humankind inappropriately interfering with the natural world or raised general concerns about unknown risks.

About three-in-ten of those who said genetic engineering of mosquitoes would be taking technology too far explained that humankind would be disrupting nature (23%) or interfering with God's plan (8%).

One respondent put it this way: "Nature is a balance and every time man interferes with it, it doesn't turn out well."

Some 24% of those with objections to the idea of reducing the fertility of mosquitoes through genetic engineering in order to reduce mosquito-borne illnesses raised concerns about the possible impact on the ecosystem.

Such responses include:

> "I do not think we know enough about the effects of removing a whole class of insects from the environment. What would be the effects on those animal and plants 'up the chain'?"

> "Mosquitoes are part of a complex ecosystem and food chain. By preventing their reproduction, we risk disrupting the entire ecosystem."

Objections to the idea of using animal biotechnology to grow organs or tissues for transplant in humans focused on beliefs about using animals for human benefit (21%) and potential risks for human health from creating human organs from animals (16%). For example:

> "In manufacturing organs, the existence of these animals would be miserable … in order to cultivate such organs the animals would need to be in a lab setting and would more than likely never see the light of day. I can't ethically say that I would agree with such a practice."
>
> "When you mix human and nonhuman genetics I believe that will cause extreme problems down the road."
>
> "Animal organs are not made for humans even though some animal and human organs may be very similar. Who knows what side effects this could cause? Even human-to-human organ transplants often reject, so I can only imagine the bad side effects that an animal-to-human transplant would cause. Keep things simple and the way nature intended."

Genetic engineering could produce more nutritious meat by altering animal proteins. Those who think this is taking technology too far raised a number of different concerns. Some cited general concerns about as-yet-unknown risks (20% of those asked), while a similar share (19%) saw this as messing with nature or God's plan in a way that goes beyond what humans should do.

One respondent put it this way: "Should we as human beings change the course of nature's 'natural selection' and potentially introduce unintended serious consequences?"

About one-in-ten (12%) objected to the idea on the grounds that people should rely less on meat in their diet or that any genetic engineering in foods is a likely health risk.

One example of these concerns: "Meat is nutritious as it is. There is no need to try to increase nutrition. Rather we should be decreasing human reliance on meat as a foodstuff."

Those who objected to the idea of bringing back extinct species often raised concerns about unintended harm to the ecosystem. Roughly two-in-ten (18%) of those asked explained their views by saying there is a reason that these animals are currently extinct, with some saying these animals would be unlikely to survive if brought back, and another 12% of this group raised potential risks to other species and the ecosystem from bringing an extinct animal into a different world.

For example:

> "Beware of unintended consequences. The universe is in balance with them extinct. Consider the problems man has created by reintroducing species that have become extinct [in] a given area, i.e., wolves and mountain lions to areas now occupied by humans and domestic livestock."

Others discussed these ideas in terms of God's plan and human interference with the natural world (23%).

A few examples:

> "God is the creator of all living things, not mankind. Extinction is part of evolution of the universe."
>
> "Nature has selected species to become extinct over millions and millions of years. We have no right to bring animals back and play God."

And 14% said they regard bringing back an extinct species as taking technology too far because they do not see a need or purpose to this, especially as it does not seem to bring any benefit to humans, or that resources should be focused elsewhere.

Objections to genetic engineering of aquarium fish raise questions about need, benefit

A sampling of these concerns:

> "For what purpose would it be done? Is there a benefit to humanity other than having a rare zoo specimen? Would

> the extinct species cease to become extinct through natural reproduction—if not that, the whole effort is without merit."
>
> "I don't see the purpose of bringing any animal back. Would it provide a better way of life for humans?"

Objections to the idea of changing the appearance of aquarium fish using genetic engineering to make the fish glow often focused on the lack of apparent need or benefit to either humans or animals.

About half (48%) of those who say engineering a glowing fish takes technology too far said they do not see the purpose for humans or society, questioned its necessity or considered it frivolous or a waste of resources.

Some examples:

> "… [While] changing a fish to glow might sound like something people would want to see it's not something beneficial to humankind. At this point it would just [be] playing God to entertain rather [than] help us."
>
> "It's frivolous. Technology should be used to help people, animals and the environment, not put on a glow show."
>
> "Why? If you only do something because you can is not a good reason. If any genetic engineering is allowed it will get out of hand. It would be a fine line that I am sure we would cross."
>
> "It seems a frivolous thing to do, much like someone getting plastic surgery to remove wrinkles or other signs of aging. The person's life is not extended by a 'better' appearance. The aquarium fish also do not benefit from their changed appearance."

Viewpoint 4

> *"Powerful genome editing techniques, it has been proposed, might be used to change animal traits in ways that benefit both them and us."*

Genome Editing Might Improve Animal Welfare, but It's Not That Simple

Anna Wilkinson

In the following viewpoint, Anna Wilkinson explores the issues raised as the UK debates new post-EU agriculture policies. The author points out that editing livestock has not garnered the attention other genetic engineering issues have. And she argues that while many applications of genetic engineering could increase animal welfare, the situation is more complex than it might at first seem. Anna Wilkinson is programme officer for the Nuffield Council on Bioethics.

As you read, consider the following questions:

1. What differences does the author distinguish between selective breeding and genome editing?
2. How might genome editing increase animal welfare, according to the viewpoint?
3. What harms can technology pose to animals?

"Genome Editing to Improve Farmed Animal Welfare. What's Not to Like?" by Anna Wilkinson, Nuffield Council on Bioethics, February 19, 2020. Reprinted by permission.

At the start of the month the Government's Agriculture Bill, which will legislate for policies to replace the EU's Common Agricultural Policy following the UK's departure from the EU, passed its second reading.

Now in the committee stage, MPs are in the process of conducting a detailed examination of the Bill's provisions that will set out the UK's future approach to farming. One of the areas currently under scrutiny is the Bill's implications for livestock farming and, particularly, animal welfare.

The welfare of farmed animals is not just topical because of the Agriculture Bill. In scientific circles there is increasing interest in the ways in which new molecular tools might be used to reduce the negative impacts of farming on animals. Powerful genome editing techniques, it has been proposed, might be used to change animal traits in ways that benefit both them and us. The idea is that animals might as a result be subjected to fewer painful procedures, be made immune to certain diseases or rendered less sensitive to extremes of hot and cold environments. People have even proposed creating animals that feel no pain.

Most of these ideas are already taking shape in the lab. Yet somewhat surprisingly, the fact that researchers have been creating genetically hornless cows, pigs resistant to the common and devastating PRRS virus, chickens resistant to avian flu, and cows that are tolerant to heat has hit the headlines relatively rarely. Whilst the ethical issues raised by heritable human genome editing (of which there is currently only one known real world instance) have inspired reams of column inches, the issues raised by editing livestock have gone relatively undiscussed in the media, civil society and the public.

Use of genetic interventions in animal agriculture, it should be noted, would not be new. In fact, the development of genome editing applications would continue a line of genetic technologies, including whole genome sequencing, which use analysis of individual animals' genetic information to enable selection of the "best" animals for breeding. Genome editing now offers the

Gene-Edited Animals Will Intensify the Climate Crisis and Could Harm Human Health

A new report from Friends of the Earth and Logos Environmental reveals that the use of gene editing in farm animals poses risks to human health, the environment and animal welfare. The report comes on the heels of research by the FDA showing that gene-edited hornless cattle have unexpected antibiotic resistant genes, despite researchers' original claims that they did not contain any genetic errors. This new report sheds light on the unintended consequences of gene editing and considers the implications for U.S. regulations.

Many genetically engineered farm animals are currently in development, funded by private companies or governments and enabled by new gene editing technologies such as CRISPR. Examples include super-muscly cows and pigs, hornless cattle, chickens and pigs made to resist certain diseases, cows with human genes, and other genetic experiments. Production of these gene-edited farm animals is often done with little public awareness or input.

"The scientific evidence shows that gene editing, particularly in animals, is far from 'precise.' Instead, it can produce unintended

opportunity to take things one step further. Rather than simply selecting from a pool of existing animals, genome editing allows breeders to directly alter animal genomes, potentially creating new traits not found in existing breeds.

There is debate about the significance of the distinction between changing the characteristic genomes of species over time through selection, and making changes by use of molecular techniques to directly alter animal genomes. Whether there is any real ethical difference between the two, as well as how this might overlap with questions about "animal nature," is hotly contested and one of the many issues that we are considering in the Nuffield Council's current inquiry into the ethical issues raised by genome editing in farmed animals, which is due to conclude at the end of 2020.

changes to genetic material and disrupt genetic processes. Such effects could have far reaching consequences for food safety, so these applications will require a rigorous assessment if they are to be used in agriculture," said co-author Dr. Janet Cotter of Logos Environmental.

"Corporate profits are a major motivation behind these genetic experiments, and we should be wary of proposals for gene-edited farm animals," said Dana Perls, report co-author and senior food and technology campaigner with Friends of the Earth. "The types of genetically engineered animals being developed will exacerbate the polluting factory farm model of agriculture and put more money in the hands of climate-destroying Big Ag. We need sustainable and ecological agriculture systems that support the health of animals, preserve and restore biodiversity and protect public health."

The new report compiles evidence from peer-reviewed scientific studies demonstrating research gaps and unknown and unintended consequences of gene editing in animals. For example, published studies have found enlarged tongues in engineered rabbits and extra vertebrae in pigs, as the *Wall Street Journal* reported in 2018. Recent cell studies linked CRISPR to DNA damage and cancer concerns.

"Gene-Edited Animals Will Intensify Factory Farming and the Climate Crisis, Could Harm Human Health," Friends of the Earth, September 17, 2019.

One real, if contingent, difference between selective breeding and the genome editing applications currently in development concerns the purposes for which they're designed. Whilst either approach could be used for a range of reasons, it so happens that selective breeding has historically been used mainly to enhance yields by increasing growth rate, muscle mass, and milk or egg production. On the other hand, the most prominent genome editing applications in development are ones that purport to produce significant animal welfare benefits.

Take polled cattle—genetically hornless cows—an application being developed by Acceligen, a subsidiary of the American biotech company Recombinetics, and compare it with what the technology might replace. The physical removal of cows' horns in order to minimise harm to other animals and farm workers is common practice in cattle farming. This can be done either by dehorning (by sawing or cutting) or disbudding (removing calves' horn buds before any horn material is visible). Both procedures can be painful for animals and, in adult cows, dehorning has been associated with prolonged wound healing, infection and increased risks of sinusitis.

Another example: Porcine Reproductive and Respiratory Syndrome (PRRS), common in farmed pigs, causes a range of unpleasant symptoms, affects reproduction, and gives rise to respiratory tract illness in young animals that can result in death. There is no effective vaccine or treatment for PRRS so a disease resistance genome editing application—currently being developed by Genus in collaboration with the Roslin Institute—appears to be the only viable prospect for fully protecting animals from the virus.

Another proposed application of genome editing would enable fetal sexing of layer chickens (birds bred specifically to lay eggs) before eggs hatch, preventing the birth, and immediate destruction, of male chicks that, of course, could not produce eggs. Live maceration is reportedly the fate of six billion one-day-old chicks each year.

So described, these interventions sound uniformly positive: what objection could anyone who cares about animal welfare possibly make? But, as is often the case with the technological innovation, things are not quite this simple.

One concern relates to possible knock-on effects on the environments in which livestock are reared. If animals are made immune to certain diseases, for example, this might affect the stocking densities at which they can be housed. The increased risks of disease spreading in more crowded groups provides (helpfully, some might argue) a "natural" limit on the degree to which they can be productively farmed in very close quarters. If this risk were reduced or removed altogether then it might be easier to pack more animals together in crowded spaces. Not necessarily a win for proponents of animal welfare. Something similar might apply to hornless cows or tailless pigs, where head butting or tail biting might otherwise be addressed by providing more space for cows or more straw for pigs.

A broader issue with high-tech welfare interventions concerns the extent to which we should be aiming to improve the lives of farmed animals at all, a question which ties in with an older debate between those arguing for animal welfare and those that defend animal rights. There is a line of thought amongst some animal rights theorists that initiatives to improve animal welfare have the effect of sanitising and legitimising uses of animals that are in principle wrong. This would make those welfare initiatives, odd as it might seem, themselves wrong. If intensive farming systems should be radically reeled in or stopped altogether (as those who argue for the abolition of animal farming contest) there would be a problem with genome editing for welfare if the result would be to perpetuate and prolong use of these systems. So even if genome editing were to confer net welfare benefits on animals that exist in these systems now, it might still be problematic.

This argument has a parallel in the broader discussion about food systems and the future of farming more generally. A widely held view in food policy and academia is that existing animal agriculture systems are, in a range of ways, giving rise to a great many negative impacts on the environment and human beings, as well as on animals. We might then need to rethink the way we produce food globally. Given that the aims of many welfare-oriented genome editing applications are to mitigate the effects on animals of larger, intensive systems, the likes of which we have many other reasons to reign in or even phase out, we should perhaps be directing our research and policy resources elsewhere. Should we be replacing these systems rather than sticking a genome editing shaped band-aid on them?

None of these issues are straightforward, of course. The likely animal welfare implications, like the wider social, economic and environmental implications, of different genome editing applications will be complex and hard to gauge. In the UK, animal welfare standards are high relative to global standards so existing regulation and law might prevent or constrain any unintended negative impacts on animals (though effects in other parts of the world might be less certain). And the extent to which we should be judging genome editing by different standards to those that have seen the widespread use of selective breeding technologies, not to mention vaccines and veterinary medicine, in livestock for many decades is a further question. These things all need to be thought about.

But when we do think about this, and when considering my original question—what's not to like?—we need to remember to think not only about the animals in front of us, but about animal agriculture more broadly and the wider context in which these debates are taking place. The challenge with genome editing livestock for welfare is to think about how the great potential of these technologies might be realised in ways that benefit animals without undermining broader efforts to make animal farming less harmful to animals, less damaging to the environment and, as a result, better for everyone. As the Agriculture Bill progresses and other agricultural policy and regulation is developed following the UK's departure from the EU, these questions should be central to working out the UK's future approach to farming.

Viewpoint 5

> *"The majority of work on genetically modified farm animals is still in the research phase and is yet to be used commercially."*

The Ethics of Genetically Modifying Farm Animals Is Still a Work in Progress

YourGenome

In the following viewpoint, authors from YourGenome examine the use of genetic modification in farm animals more closely. The viewpoint poses some basic questions about the ethics of genetically modifying farm animals and offers answers from both sides of the issue. YourGenome is a website that offers information and education about DNA, genes, and genomes.

As you read, consider the following questions:

1. What examples of harm to animals due to genetic engineering do the authors give?
2. What examples of benefits are listed here?
3. What did the UK's Animal Welfare Act require?

"Is It Ethical to Genetically Modify Farm Animals for Agriculture?" yourgenome.org, https://www.yourgenome.org/debates/is-it-ethical-to-genetically-modify-farm-animals-for-agriculture.

The number of genetically modified animals used in agriculture has increased significantly in recent years. Researchers have genetically engineered a number of mammals, from laboratory animals to farm animals, as well as birds, fish and insects.

The most widely used genetically modified animals are laboratory animals, such as the fruitfly (*Drosophila*) and mice. Genetically engineered animals enable scientists to gain an insight into basic biological processes and the relationships between mutations and disease.

However, farm animals, such as sheep, goats and cows, can also be genetically modified to enhance specific characteristics. These can include milk production and disease resistance, as well as improving the nutritional value of the products they are farmed for. For example, cows, goats and sheep have been genetically engineered to express specific proteins in their milk.

The majority of work on genetically modified farm animals is still in the research phase and is yet to be used commercially. Below are some of the advantages and disadvantages associated with genetically modifying animals for agriculture, divided up into four key areas:

1. Do the benefits of genetically modified farm animals outweigh the risks?
2. Is genetic modification of farm animals ethical?
3. Is it morally acceptable to genetically modify farm animals?
4. Is there a thorough regulatory process for genetic modification of farm animals?

Do the Benefits of Genetically Modified Farm Animals Outweigh the Risks?

Yes

Genetic engineering holds great potential in many fields, including agriculture, medicine and industry.

Genetic modification can increase the yield from farm animals, for example cows can be engineered to produce more milk for the same size of herd.

Genetically modified farm animals are being used to produce important medicinal products, such as antibodies, in large quantities. These products can be used for the treatment of many different human conditions. The current production system for such products is donated human blood, which is in limited supply due to a lack of donors.

Sheep and goats can be modified to produce medicinal products in their milk. This has no negative impact on the animal but the product can help to treat human diseases.

No

The transfer of genetic material from one species to another raises potentially serious health issues for animals and humans.

There is a risk that new diseases from genetically engineered animals could be spread to non-genetically engineered animals, and even humans.

In many cases, selective breeding is just as effective as genetic engineering and doesn't carry the same risks.

We don't yet know if eating the products of genetically modified animals could potentially harm us.

Is Genetic Modification of Farm Animals Ethical?

Yes

Genetic engineering is a logical continuation of selective breeding, which has been done by humans for thousands of years.

Genetic engineering of animals is strictly controlled by animal cruelty legislations in many countries and is always carefully scrutinised by teams of experts before being approved for wider use.

No

Many of the embryos that undergo genetic engineering procedures do not survive.

Genetic modification can put animals at risk of harm. For example, transgenic pigs were found to be arthritic, partially blind and infertile when a human growth hormone was inserted into their genomes to make them grow faster.

Is It Morally Acceptable to Genetically Modify Farm Animals?

Yes

Not all genetic engineering directly benefits humans. Some genetic engineering is to improve resistance of livestock to disease, for example, bovine spongiform encephalopathy ("mad cow disease") in cattle. It can also be used to remove characteristics that cause injury, for example, selecting for cattle without horns.

Animals have been used to help humans for millennia. Many would say that human lives are of higher moral value than animal lives.

The percentage of genetically modified farm animals is tiny compared to the number of animals slaughtered for humans to eat. This practice is widely seen as morally acceptable.

No

Research could use other organisms such as plants and bacteria to mass produce therapies for human medicine. For example, genetically engineered cereal grains to produce human proteins.

The cost to the animal always outweighs the benefits as, by carrying out genetic engineering, we are violating their rights.

Genetic engineering often involves modifying animals for reasons that have no benefit for that species, and could potentially cause them pain and discomfort.

We shouldn't be attempting to "play God." Life should not be regarded as a product that can be altered and played with for economic benefit.

Is There a Thorough Regulatory Process for Genetic Modification of Farm Animals?

Yes

It has been suggested that, as a rule, genetically engineered animals should be no worse off than the equivalent stock would be if they were not genetically engineered.

The Animal Welfare Act, a federal law passed in the UK in 1966, requires all entities looking to carry out research with animals to have their programme reviewed before they go ahead, have veterinary care programmes in place and staff that are qualified to care for live animals.

The UK Home Office Animals (Scientific Procedures) Act 1986 has set out guidelines for research involving animals.

The FDA (Food and Drug Administration) in the USA regulates genetic engineering with animals and their products under the new animal drug provisions of the Federal Food, Drug and Cosmetic Act (FFDCA). It helps monitor and maintain certain standards, including input from the public, when it comes to genetically engineering animals.

The "new animal drug" provisions of the FFDCA focuses on whether the new animal drug is safe for the animal and if it is effective. If the drug is for a food-producing animal it also focuses on whether the resulting food is safe to eat.

No

Genetic engineering of animals is a relatively new practice and is mainly used in research. As a result regulations for its use in farming are minimal.

For regulations that have been put in place for the use of animals in research, it is often unclear how they would be applied to genetic engineering of farm animals and few guidelines refer to it directly.

Periodical and Internet Sources Bibliography

The following articles have been selected to supplement the diverse views presented in this chapter.

Gregory Barber, "A More Humane Livestock Industry, Brought to You by CRISPR," *Wired*, March 19, 2019, https://www.wired.com/story/crispr-gene-editing-humane-livestock/.

Vittoria D'Alessio, "We Need to Talk About CRISPR," *Horizon*, December 17, 2019, https://ec.europa.eu/research-and-innovation/en/horizon-magazine/we-need-talk-about-crispr.

Pallab Ghosh, "Gene Edited Farm Animals Are on Their Way," BBC News, June 20, 2018, https://www.bbc.com/news/science-environment-44388038.

Veronique Greenwood, "How CRISPR Is Spreading Through the Animal Kingdom," *Nova*, May 23, 2018, https://www.pbs.org/wgbh/nova/article/crispr-animals/.

Kristin Houser, "China Isn't Afraid to Be the 'Bad Guy' of CRISPR Research: And the World Could Reap the Benefits from Disease Cures to Ending World Hunger," Futurism, July 31, 2019, https://futurism.com/china-bad-guy-crispr-research.

Blake Hurst, "CRISPR Will Make GMOs Ubiquitous," *National Review*, March 19, 2018, https://www.nationalreview.com/2018/03/crispr-will-make-gmos-ubiquitous/.

Carolyn Y. Johnson, "Gene-Edited Farm Animals Are Coming. Will We Eat Them?" *Washington Post*, December 17, 2018, https://www.washingtonpost.com/news/national/wp/2018/12/17/feature/gene-edited-farm-animals-are-coming-will-we-eat-them/.

David Lawrence, "Genetic Engineering and Human-Animal Hybrids: How China Is Leading a Global Split in Controversial Research," The Conversation, September 3, 2019, https://theconversation.com/genetic-engineering-and-human-animal-hybrids-how-china-is-leading-a-global-split-in-controversial-research-121473.

Michael Le Page, "Cattle Are Being Gene Edited to Help Them Survive Climate Change," *New Scientist*, October 5, 2020, https://www.newscientist.com/article/2256097-cattle-are-being-gene-edited-to-help-them-survive-climate-change/.

Megan Thielking and Andrew Joseph, "A Giant Gorilla and a Winged Wolf: Does Rampage Get the Science of CRISPR Right?" Stat News, April 12, 2018, https://www.statnews.com/2018/04/12/crispr-monster-animals-rampage-review/.

OPPOSING VIEWPOINTS® SERIES

Chapter 3

Should We Genetically Modify Animals to Replace Extinct Animals?

Chapter Preface

In previous chapters, viewpoint authors discussed the use of gene-editing technology to cure human illnesses, improve food production and nutrition, and possibly make the lives of livestock less stressful. In this chapter, viewpoints turn to a very different use of this remarkable new technology: de-extinction.

De-extinction is a process that would use DNA from extinct species, along with similar living animals, to create a new creature that is very much like—if not quite identical to—an extinct species. No one can deny that bringing back a woolly mammoth or a dodo bird would be super cool. (Sorry, but it won't work with dinosaurs; they're too old.) However, proponents of this technology say that it is far more than that. The reason for resurrecting these animals is not just to gawk at them. It's to reintroduce them to habitats they once lived in. The hope is that returning species to these habitats will save entire ecosystems and thereby save many other species from extinction.

For many years, the idea seemed quixotic at best. But CRISPR technology has brought de-extinction tantalizingly close to reality. Now science and society are grappling with the potential consequences and implications of de-extinction. Could the technology help restore not only individual species but entire ecosystems? Could the lessons learned from this new science help advance science in important ways? Even if we never see a woolly mammoth or a dodo bird, would the science itself be worth the investment?

Or are the risks of such a transformative technology just too great? Do we know enough about the complex interactions of ecosystems to interfere with them in such a dramatic way? The viewpoint authors in this chapter take on these questions and more.

VIEWPOINT 1

> *"We also have to ask ourselves how much we care about these problems and whether or not we're willing to take risks."*

Genetic Engineering Could Save Our Planet's Biodiversity

Andrew Moore

People working on de-extinction projects often claim that genetic engineering could help restore biodiversity to the planet. In the following viewpoint, Andrew Moore reports on research that aims to use genetic engineering not to bring back extinct species, but to alter existing ones in ways that could protect them from threats and make them more resilient. Andrew Moore is marketing and communications manager in the College of Natural Resources at North Carolina State University.

As you read, consider the following questions:

1. What are gene drives, and how are they being used in the research discussed in this viewpoint?
2. Why does Jason Delborne say that this research must not be conducted behind closed doors?
3. What are the risks of deploying altered animals into existing ecosystems?

A U.N. report published last month painted a stark picture of global biodiversity loss, estimating that more than 1 million species are at risk of extinction—many of them within decades—due to farming, logging and other human activities.

While conservationists have been successful in restoring some species, such as the southern white rhino and American bison, the average risk of extinction for birds, mammals, amphibians and corals shows no sign of decreasing.

But what if it were possible to protect our planet's biodiversity by rewriting the genetic code of plants and animals? It might sound like science fiction, but researchers at NC State's College of Natural Resources—and around the world—are considering ways to employ genetic engineering for conservation purposes, from eradicating invasive rodents on islands to increasing the resilience of American chestnut trees to an invasive fungus.

"New tools for gene editing and strategies such as synthetic gene drives open up novel opportunities for imagining ways that we might 'engineer' biology beyond laboratories and agricultural fields," said Jason Delborne, an associate professor in the Department of Forestry and Environmental Resources. "The conservation community, in particular, has begun to wrestle with whether, and how, genetic technologies might be applied to complex and challenging environmental problems."

Delborne, who is also a research leader in the Genetic Engineering and Society Center at NC State, studies the interactions between policymakers, scientists and the public, particularly in the context of emerging biotechnologies.

He is also a member of the IUCN Task Force on Synthetic Biology and Biodiversity Conservation. The international group of scientists recently published an in-depth assessment of genetic engineering and its potential impacts on conservation.

We sat down with Delborne, who co-authored several of the report's chapters, to find out all there is to know about genetic engineering, from the basics of how it works to whether or not it can actually help solve our planet's biodiversity crisis.

A New Tool for Conservation

Genetic engineering is the process of manipulating or altering the genetic makeup of an organism—be it an animal, plant or a bacterium. This can be achieved by using biotechnology to remove a gene from one organism and inserting it into another, giving it the ability to express the trait encoded by that gene.

Humans have been manipulating life for thousands of years. In fact, many of today's domesticated plants and animals are a result of selective breeding, which involves choosing organisms with desirable traits and mating them in hopes that their offspring inherit those traits. One of the best known examples is the modern dog, which was the first species to be selectively bred and domesticated by humans from Eurasian gray wolves at least 15,000 years ago.

By the mid-20th century, genetic engineering became more widely recognized as a specific and distinct field of science, with researchers not only identifying the structure of DNA but also developing methods of manipulating it.

Researchers have since developed new technologies that allow more precise and targeted changes to an organism's DNA, such as CRISPR and other gene editing methods. These technologies also make it theoretically possible to transmit changes across an entire breeding population, even in the wild, through the use of gene drives.

Gene drives are tiny snippets of DNA that have been tweaked by scientists to alter the way that certain genes (and therefore traits) are inherited. Normally, a gene has a 50-50 chance of being passed from parent to offspring. Gene drives increase that probability to upwards of 95 percent. Some conservationists are considering ways to use this technology to help protect threatened or endangered species.

Delborne, for instance, is working with an international consortium of scientists, including several other NC State researchers, to study the potential use of gene drives to eradicate invasive rodents from oceanic islands. Often brought aboard sealing and whaling ships in the 19th century, these rodents have swarmed the islands and wreaked ecological havoc by preying on ground-nesting seabirds and their eggs, some of which are threatened or endangered.

The consortium, known as the Genetic Biocontrol of Invasive Rodents program, is exploring the possibility of introducing modified mice on islands to breed with their wild counterparts, spreading a gene drive that ensures their offspring are male. The lack of females would theoretically cause an invasive population to crash over the course of several generations, but the technology is still years away from being deployed in the field.

The Promises and Perils of Genetics

While gene drives and other biotechnologies, if appropriately designed and targeted, might be useful tools for protecting threatened or endangered species from extinction, there is not yet enough information to determine how they will actually work in the wild, according to Delborne. This has left both the public and the scientific community cautious about their use and the potential impacts they might have on nature.

One of the major and widely acknowledged concerns is that gene drives could be difficult to contain once deployed, with the movement of modified organisms potentially extending beyond the specific location of the invasive species and impacting the ecological roles played by both target and non-target species, according to Delborne. Rodents, for instance, are an invasive species and pose an ecological threat to ground-nesting seabirds on islands, but they are native to other parts of the world where they may play a beneficial role in ecosystems.

Furthermore, the use of gene drives and other biotechnologies may have socio-economic effects on production and consumption patterns and impact the cultures, rights and livelihoods of local and indigenous communities, which manage, govern, reside in or depend on a large part of the world's biodiversity, according to Delborne. There are also regulatory uncertainties surrounding the implementation of these technologies.

"Genetic engineering has potential. But every intervention has risks, so we have to consider—and anticipate—the potential impacts of these technologies and how they compare to other tools we might use," Delborne said. "We also have to ask ourselves how much we care about these problems and whether or not we're willing to take risks. And if so, what will these technologies mean to people? It's not as simple as protecting a species. We have to think about the ways in which the use of these technologies might change how we experience the natural environment."

In their report, Delborne and other members of the IUCN Task Force on Synthetic Biology and Biodiversity Conservation noted that gene drive research, in particular, must be contained to experimental efforts in controlled environments until scientists have sufficient data to determine what will happen in the wild. And once these technologies are ready to be deployed, their use needs to be informed by case-by-case assessments of associated risks and benefits, guided by empirical evidence and incorporating traditional knowledge, religious and ethical values in decision-making.

The authors also called for increased collaboration between conservationists and researchers to gather scientific evidence that will inform the deployment of these technologies and for regulators to obtain the informed consent of indigenous peoples and local communities before introducing gene drives into the environment.

Delborne, a social scientist, is currently focused on stakeholder engagement, fostering meaningful dialogue and deliberation between the scientists proposing these technologies and the public, including indigenous communities. He has led stakeholder workshops about the genetically engineered American chestnut tree and the use of gene drive mice for conservation.

"I think one of the worst things we can do is conduct testing behind closed doors and then expect the public to just trust us when the time comes to deploy these technologies. That's not the best strategy," Delborne said. "It's much more promising to think about ways to be more transparent and to involve stakeholders along the way in conversations about the design and testing of these technologies."

He added that the assessment will ultimately help inform a new IUCN policy on the use of synthetic biology and engineered gene drives for conservation, which the international organization will vote on during the World Conservation Congress in June 2020. While the policy itself isn't a law, it will establish an important framework for researchers, conservationists and governments to consider in the decision-making process.

Viewpoint 2

> *"There is no way to bring back something that is 100 per cent identical to a species that went extinct a long time ago. Things that are gone are gone."*

We Can't Bring Back Extinct Species (But We Might Get a Suitable Replacement)

Chris Fitch

In the following viewpoint, Chris Fitch takes a deeper dive into the topic of de-extinction. The author talks with several scientists at the forefront of the movement and finds that by creating species that are similar to ones that have gone extinct, they may be able to restore the ecosystems these animals played a key role in maintaining. Chris Fitch is a travel and science writer, former staff writer at Geographical, *the magazine of the Royal Geographical Society, and the author of three books.*

As you read, consider the following questions:

1. What are keystone species, and why are they important to ecosystems?
2. Dinosaurs are off the table, writes Fitch, but how far back can de-extinction go?
3. If they have the DNA, why can't scientists bring back the exact animal that went extinct?

"Back to Life: The World of De-extinction," by Chris Fitch, Geographical Ltd., February 17, 2017. Reprinted by permission.

The passenger pigeon was a legendary species. Flying in unfathomably large numbers across North America, with potentially many millions within a single flock, their migration was once one of nature's great spectacles. The 18th century ornithologist Alexander Wilson described a flock of passing passenger pigeons as "a column, eight or ten miles in length" and on a separate occasion, claims he mistook a flock for "a tornado, about to overwhelm the house and everything around in destruction." Thousands of birds would roost together in tree branches.

John Lawson, the 17th century explorer, naturalist and writer, once noted that a flock had "broke down the limbs of a great many trees all over the woods," while numerous accounts describe trees being toppled by the weight of birds nestling among their branches. There also exist records of terrified villagers fleeing for their lives, with flocks of transiting passenger pigeons "blotting out the rays of the sun."

"For me, that's an adrenaline rush," says geneticist Ben Novak. "I want to see a biological entity that has the power to create weather. We don't have that today, we have nothing that powerful."

Sadly, the remarkable passenger pigeon's existence came to an end on 1 September 1914, when "Martha," the last living *Ectopistes migratorius*, died at Cincinnati Zoo. While estimates of passenger pigeon populations from the 19th century range from three billion to as many as ten billion individuals (with the species believed to have once constituted 25 per cent of the total bird population of the United States), they were hunted to death around the turn of the 20th century (an "industrial-scale harvest," according to Novak). A few stragglers kept the species alive in captivity, before Martha finally breathed her last.

Novak is Lead Researcher on the Great Passenger Pigeon Comeback, an ambitious project, started in 2012, which aims to bring the passenger pigeon back to life through an ambitious-sounding process commonly known as "de-extinction." Despite how much it sounds like science fiction, de-extinction is, in principle, a genuine and legitimate concept. The basic premise involves using cloning technology (such as that which famously brought us Dolly the sheep two decades ago) to turn the DNA of extinct animals into a fertilised embryo, which can be carried by a surrogate—whatever the nearest living relative is—before being born as a living, breathing animal.

For the Great Passenger Pigeon Comeback, the plan is to use the living and abundant band-tailed pigeon as a surrogate parent for passenger pigeon embryos. "It's the closest living relative, and it's ecologically very similar," explains Novak. Then, once the pregnancy has come to term, and the band-tailed surrogate has laid her eggs, they would hatch into the first living passenger pigeon chicks in over a century. "It's a very simple goal," he claims. "We want to recreate passenger pigeons, and put them back out in the wild."

Repopulation

Passenger pigeons are one of the pioneering species in this field, but they are far from the only ones on which this cutting-edge technology is being trialled. From the Pyrenean ibex to the auroch, the heath hen to the gastric-brooding frog, the de-extinction movement is stirring the imaginations of scientists around the world to consider which species could potentially make a return from the void.

In Australia, the thylacine (more commonly known as the Tasmanian tiger) is another extinct creature that genetic scientists are striving to bring back to life. Forced to compete with dingoes for food and survival, driven onto the island of Tasmania, then decimated by hunters upon the arrival of Europeans in the early 1800s, the tragic story of the thylacine, which currently ends with the death of the final individual in Hobart Zoo in 1936, could take a dramatic twist if Michael Archer, Professor at the School of Biological, Earth and Environmental Sciences, UNSW, gets his way. By scouring museum specimens, Archer and colleagues have collected DNA from a range of sources, with attempts to remove any contaminants (such as human DNA) and then successfully sequence the thylacine genome ongoing.

There are a number of criteria that Revive & Restore (a non-profit subsidiary of the Long Now Foundation, with the assigned mission to "enhance biodiversity through the genetic rescue of endangered and extinct species") has established that should be fulfilled before attempting de-extinction. The first of these asks, understandably, how possible it would actually be. Despite the hopes of many (and probably to the relief of many more), bringing back dinosaurs is off the table since their DNA is many millions of years too old to have survived intact and therefore be able to be sequenced effectively.

However, rough estimates place the length of time that can have elapsed since a species went extinct in order to be able to sequence its DNA in any significant way at around 200,000 years;

De-Extinction: The Good and the Not So Good

Benefits of De-Extinction:

- Scientific knowledge: De-extinction could offer insights into evolution and natural resources that are currently unavailable to us.
- Technological advancement: De-extinction could be a big step forward for genetic engineering.
- Environmental benefits: Threatened or damaged ecosystems could be restored with the help of certain now-extinct species.
- Justice: If people pushed plant and animals species into extinction, perhaps we owe it to these species to try and bring them back.
- Wonder: How cool would it be to see extinct species alive and kicking again?

Objections to De-Extinction:

- Animal welfare: People could be exploiting animals for solely human purposes, and may cause individuals of the de-extinct species harm.

a time frame that does leave open the possibility of bringing back to life another immensely popular candidate for this technology: the woolly mammoth.

George Church, Professor of Genetics at Harvard Medical School, and co-author of *Regenesis: How Synthetic Biology Will Reinvent Nature and Ourselves*, leads a team working on a project called the Woolly Mammoth Revival. "It's aimed at developing tools to test ideas that come from genome projects in general," he explains. "This one to find out what might be responsible for cold resistance, which is the main distinguishing feature between woolly mammoths and Asian elephants." By identifying which genetic traits made it possible for mammoths to survive the cold climates of the tundra, the project's ultimate goal is to repopulate the region with brand new mammoths.

- Health: Species could carry retroviruses or pathogens when brought back to life.
- Environment: De-extinct species would be alien and potentially invasive; their habitats and food sources have changed, so their roles in these changed ecosystems could be too.
- Political: De-extinction may change priorities in other fields of science, such as medical research and the conservation of currently endangered species.
- Moral: Is de-extinction playing god, or just plain wrong? It may also have unforeseen consequences.

If an extinct animal were brought back to life in the lab, the authors point out that it would still lack many of a species' key characteristics, such as epigenetics, environment and social groups. Plus it would bring along with it a number of complicated legalities relating to the Endangered Species Act and patent laws. And that doesn't even get into the messy world of if and how such resurrections should be regulated.

In the end, both papers seem to draw open-ended conclusions. But if the practice is really as inevitable as it seems, the authors say the most interesting part will be seeing how humanity reacts.

"5 Reasons to Bring Back Extinct Animals (And 5 Reasons Not To)," by Breanna Draxler, *Discover Magazine*, April 5, 2013.

"In a way we're ready today, in 2016," insists Church, "although we would like to avoid surrogates, because we don't want to interfere with the reproduction of either the African or the Asian elephant." While alternative, non-surrogate technologies are yet to be fully developed, Church suggests 2018 as a possible date when cloning attempts could begin.

Hybridisation

All this begs the question, if extinct species can be brought back to life, can humanity begin to correct much of the damage enacted upon the natural world over the past few millennia? "The idea of de-extinction is that we can reverse this process, bringing species that no longer exist back to life," says Beth Shapiro, Director of Evolutionary Genomics at the University of California Santa Cruz's Genomics Institute, and author of *How to Clone a Mammoth: The Science of De-Extinction*. "I don't think that we can do this. There is no way to bring back something that is 100 per cent identical to a species that went extinct a long time ago. Things that are gone are gone."

The harsh reality, as Shapiro points out, is that despite the vast improvements made with this technology, the moment a species has become extinct, the reality of bringing that exact same species back to life is basically zero. "In order to clone something, you need a living cell," she explains. "So as soon as something has been dead for a long time, there is no living cell."

Instead, for de-extinction as we understand it to work, the DNA of existing species needs to be used as a template, ready for the insertion of strands of extinct animal DNA to create something new; a hybrid of two species, based on the living species, but which looks and/or acts like the animal which died out.

This is broadly the same process which has taken place in countless "de-extinction" projects. The passenger pigeon embryo that could potentially be placed inside a band-tailed surrogate parent would be formed through the editing of band-tailed pigeon DNA to include characteristics that are similar to that of the passenger pigeon. "We're actually re-writing the genome code, so that it carries the mutations of a passenger pigeon," explains Ben Novak.

Similarly, attempts to recreate the lost auroch involve the selective sampling of DNA from several existing "primitive" breeds of cattle, while Revive & Restore's Heath Hen Project significantly utilises the genetic code of the extinct heath hen's closest living relative, the greater prairie chicken.

"We'll never find a living mammoth cell, for example," explains Shapiro. "Instead, you would have to take an elephant cell, like George Church's group are doing, and edit that into a mammoth."

While Asian elephants happen to be genetically even closer to extinct mammoths than they are to living African elephants, the differences between the two are still substantial, and geneticists remain a long way from being able to alter all million and a half base pairs in the genetic code, which would turn an Asian elephant cell into a genetically accurate mammoth cell.

Furthermore, even in the rare cases in which DNA can be extracted and sequenced to the point that an animal could be created with all the A, C, G and T nucleobases in the right places, there would remain the massively complicated challenge of teaching animals with no natural parents, conceived and born in entirely controlled circumstances, often by people who have never seen a real life individual before, how to behave like the extinct animal they are trying to bring back to life.

"We have little way to know how mammoth-like versus elephant-like this animal would be," continues Shapiro. "They're going to be born and raised by elephants, they're going to eat an elephant diet, they're going to establish in their guts an elephant microbiome. It's got to be taught how to be a living, breathing, adult social animal by an elephant, not by a mammoth. So, is it going to be a mammoth, or is it going to be an elephant?"

Ecological Niches

This complicated process and questionable outcome begs the question: what is the actual point of this technology? If true passenger pigeons, mammoths and countless other extinct animals remain, despite our best efforts, lost from nature's family tree forever, then what are the logical motivations behind continuing this field of research?

One leading argument is that the dramatic and relatively recent loss of many species, particularly in the past century, has left several ecological niches unfilled, gaps which we are only recently coming to understand as being somewhat pivotal to the health of the wider ecosystem.

"There is no carnivore now in Tasmania that fills the niche which thylacines once occupied," explains Michael Archer. He points out that the years since the thylacine went extinct has seen a trophic cascade whereby the lack of competition for Tasmanian devils—the island's other notorious resident—has seen the spread of the "dangerously debilitating" facial tumour syndrome, which threatens the very existence of Tasmanian devils themselves. "If that contagious cancer had popped up previously, it would have burned out in whatever region it started. The return of thylacines to Tasmania could help to ensure that devils are never again put at risks of this kind."

Furthermore, the purpose of recreating the passenger pigeon isn't simply because of a wish to witness flocks of birds blocking out the sun. "For us, the goal has always been replacing these extinct species with a suitable replacement," explains Novak. "Band-tailed pigeons are fiercely territorial breeders. When it comes to breeding, they scatter, and make maybe one or two nests per hectare. Whereas passenger pigeons, they're very social. When they would roost, they would make 10,000 or more nests in one hectare. That disturbance in the forest, that's actually the ecological role that the passenger pigeon played, and nothing alive today can really re-assume that role."

In the absence of such a keystone species, ecosystems in the eastern US have suffered, as the lack of disturbance of thousands of passenger pigeons wrecking trees and branches means there has been minimal need for regrowth, leaving forests stagnant and therefore unwelcoming to the plants and animals that evolved to help regenerate the forest after a disturbance. A hybridised band-tailed pigeon, with the added nesting habits of a passenger pigeon, could, in theory, reestablish that forest disturbance, and thereby create the diverse habitat necessary for many plants, insects, mammals and other native species to thrive. In those terms, Novak sees highlighting the difference between genuine and hybridised species as just "nitpicking."

As well as his principle role on the passenger pigeon project, Novak is also in the very early stages of investigating the possibility of bringing back to the island of Mauritius possibly the world's most famously extinct animal, the dodo, which, as he points out, is basically just a giant pigeon.

"All of the technology developed for passenger pigeons can be leveraged for a dodo bird project," he explains. "There might be an ecological importance to a dodo on that island, partly because of how big it is. It's got one of the biggest mouths of the endemic fauna, so it's capable of eating a class of fruits and seeds that other species were not eating. So its role as a key seed disperser is important."

While there is a consensus that there is little habitat left in which a new dodo species could survive, there is an argument that the interest generated by the potential return of the dodo would provide essential funding. This would go a long way towards speeding up the habitat restoration and removal of invasive species needed on Mauritius both for potential dodos, and, crucially, for living endangered species. "A dodo bird project could really take off, and hopefully the people of Mauritius think so as well," he smiles.

"Thinking about things in terms of species is not really the right way think about it," argues Shapiro. "If you're just going to get an elephant, have you really brought a mammoth back to life? I think the answer to that depends on your motivation for doing this. If you want to bring a mammoth back to life because you want to put it in a zoo or you think it's cool to be able to bring something back that's dead, then you've failed. If you want to bring something back that maybe is able to fill the niche of a mammoth, then you just need an elephant that can live where mammoths once lived. That is a much more compelling reason to think about de-extinction, in terms of what we can do to help preserve ecosystems, to re-establish functional ecosystems, and re-establish interactions between species that are gone because species have gone extinct. I think that can be an incredibly compelling reason to think about this technology."

Genetic Rescue

While the prospect of bringing back to life extinct animals might capture imaginations, it is, of course, far easier to try to save a living, breathing species that is merely threatened with extinction. "Many of the technologies that people have in mind when they think about de-extinction can be used as a form of 'genetic rescue,'" explains Shapiro.

She prefers to focus the debate on how this emerging technology could be used to fully understand why various species went extinct in the first place, and therefore how we could use it to make genetic modifications that could prevent mass extinctions as a result of human activity and climate change in the future. "This technology—although it doesn't exist yet—could be incredibly useful as a new weapon in what should be a growing arsenal to fight contemporary extinctions," she insists.

While enabling mammoths (or mammoth-like Asian elephants) to return to the tundra and boreal forests of Eurasia and North America could be a useful factor in reducing carbon emissions—the disruptive impact of elephants punching holes through snow and knocking down trees believed to encourage grass growth, thereby increasing albedo, reducing temperatures, and mitigating emissions from melting permafrost—there is also the significant role such actions could have on the elephants themselves.

"Probably my highest priority would be preserving the endangered Asian elephant," says George Church, "expanding their range to the huge ecosystem of the tundra. It's probably the largest ecosystem in the world, and it has the lowest population density of humans." Necessary adaptations would include smaller ears, thicker hair, and extra insulating fat, all for the purpose of reducing heat loss in the tundra, and all elements contained within the genetic code of the extinct woolly mammoth.

Of course, many extinct animals wouldn't be able to survive in our contemporary environment even if they could be successfully brought back to life. Therefore, another of the Revive & Restore criteria asks why the species initially went extinct, and whether that problem has changed. Is it simply because of over-hunting, which cultural changes may have eliminated? Or are we trying to bring a species back just because it's fun "playing God"?

The latter is an accusation that geneticists such as Shapiro have had to get used to. "We are not messing with things," she counters. "We, as a species, have been manipulating and directing the evolutionary trajectory of the organisms with which we share this planet for at least the last 30,000 years, which is the first time we find evidence in the archaeological record of grey wolves being domesticated as dogs. We're simply now asking for the capacity to do it in a more directed way."

"I would also say there's an incredible moral hazard to not do anything at all," she continues. "We know that what we are doing today is not enough, and we have to be willing to take some calculated and measured risks."

Matter of Time

While genuine de-extinction—the returning of 100 per cent genetically accurate extinct creatures to our environment—remains merely science fiction, the opportunities available as a result of genetic rescue technology potentially offer a difference between survival and complete extinction for many species that could only have been imagined even just a few years ago.

Furthermore, if the ultimate goal is to find a way to fill certain ecological niches that humans have left vacant, then it may not be too long before this ambition is realised for real.

"It's a matter of time and it's a matter of funding," explains Novak, who anticipates that, with the necessary financial support, a first batch of engineered birds could be hatched by 2022. "I don't think there will be many billions of passenger pigeons again," he predicts, "but we can definitely get up to the millions or hundreds of millions range, and they can block out for sun for a couple of hours again."

Viewpoint 3

> *"We have learned from biological invasions that putting new species into ecosystems can have large economic and ecological effects, sometimes positive and sometimes negative, but almost always difficult or impossible to predict or control. "*

De-Extinction Is Too Risky

David L. Strayer

Though many proponents of de-extinction and genetic engineering technology see it as a wonderful new strategy for saving ecosystems in peril, in the following viewpoint, David L. Strayer argues that the risk to existing ecosystems is too great to proceed with introducing bioengineered species to existing ecosystems. While the author agrees that the method may have promise, he contends that we need to slow down before taking steps that could have irreversible consequences. David L. Strayer is a freshwater ecologist and distinguished senior scientist at the Cary Institute for Ecosystem Studies.

"De-Extinction, a Risky Ecological Experiment," by Dave Strayer, February 19, 2016.

As you read, consider the following questions:

1. What are some examples of introductions of animals to ecosystems that backfired spectacularly?
2. How does the author suggest preparing for potential problems created by introductions of bioengineered species?
3. What argument does the author make for delaying the use of de-extinction technology?

De-extinction (bringing extinct species back from the dead) has been riding a wave of enthusiasm, fueled by Steward Brand's TED talk and several prominent books and articles. But for a project that aspires to use materials from the past to build a better future, de-extinction is doing a poor job of using past experience with biological invasions to temper that enthusiasm.

The basic idea of de-extinction is to use bits of genetic material salvaged from an extinct species (museum specimens, frozen mammoths) in cutting-edge biotechnology to create living animals in the lab, and use these lab-created specimens to re-establish populations of the extinct species in the wild. Actually, as Beth Shapiro described in her excellent book *How To Clone a Mammoth*, the end product isn't literally the extinct species, but an animal with some of the genes of the extinct species (the passenger pigeon) and some of the genes of a living relative (e.g., the band-tailed pigeon), which hopefully looks and acts something like the extinct species. We might call this new species "passenger pigeon v.2.0."

I don't need to explain the appeal of "de-extinction." Besides using our powers to bring back charismatic species, de-extinction could restore vital functions that these lost animals performed, and thus benefit other inhabitants of their ecosystems. De-extinction is also almost irresistibly cool (come on! Bringing mammoths back from the dead?).

Much of the discussion about de-extinction has focused on the technical challenges of resurrecting extinct species, the problem of choosing which species to revive, and the danger that de-extinction could divert attention and resources away from badly needed programs to prevent further extinctions. These serious problems deserve careful consideration, and are well treated in Shapiro's book and elsewhere. But focusing on these problems can distract us from what may be the central risk of de-extinction: that its ecological effects could be large, and hard to predict and manage.

We have learned from biological invasions that putting new species into ecosystems can have large economic and ecological effects, sometimes positive and sometimes negative, but almost always difficult or impossible to predict or control. Familiar examples include rabbits in Australia; or zebra mussels, emerald ash borers, and chestnut blight in the US, among many others. The combination of large effects, low predictability, and irreversibility makes putting new species into ecosystems, including de-extinction, a risky enterprise.

As for any human activity that poses risks to the environment, proponents of de-extinction should be able to provide good answers to three questions: What are its likely effects? What is the plan to prevent or repair unexpected damage? Why should this project be done now, instead of being deferred?

The usual answer to the first question is that the species is being returned to the ecosystem in which it lived for many years, and will simply resume its former ecological roles. This answer fails on two counts. First, because we've been changing our world so rapidly, a de-extinguished species won't be restored to its former ecosystem, but to a different, sometimes radically different, ecosystem. Since the passenger pigeon was last abundant, its home in eastern North America has been transformed from forests to industrial farms, superhighways, and megalopolises; its human population has increased 5-fold; we've poured huge amounts of nutrients and toxins into the landscape; thousands of species from other parts of the world have become established, while others (like American chestnut) have dwindled or disappeared; and we are in the process of changing its climate.

Ecologists know that the setting into which a species is placed strongly affects its roles and impacts, so there is no reason to expect that passenger pigeon v.2.0 (or any other de-extinguished species) would simply re-assume its former roles. Experience with native North American species like white-tailed deer, Canada geese, coyotes, and Colorado potato beetles shows that the roles that these species play (and human valuation of those roles) changed radically as ecological and societal contexts changed.

The second objection to the naïve answer that a de-extinguished species would simply resume its former roles is that v.2.0 isn't the same as the extinct species. In all but a few of the cases that are being discussed, the organism to be released won't literally be the species that was lost, but rather a human creation that in some ways looks and acts like the lost species. This match might be pretty close, or merely superficial (e.g., a cold-hardy, hairy elephant in place of a woolly mammoth). Even small differences between v.2.0 and the original could cause large differences in roles and effects.

Again, experience with biological invasions shows that this isn't just a theoretical possibility. When two similar species of sparrow were released in North America, one spread quickly and became a widespread nuisance (the house sparrow), while its cousin never left the St. Louis area or caused problems (the Eurasian tree sparrow). The example of the common reed (Phragmites) is even more striking. Native strains of this species were a widespread but minor part of North American wetlands. When nearly indistinguishable Eurasian strains were introduced, they formed impenetrable thickets all across North America, crowding out native plants, damaging wildlife habitat, and disrupting nutrient cycles. Wetlands managers now spend millions of dollars each year to burn, herbicide, mow, dig up, and otherwise kill Eurasian Phragmites in North America. Organisms that look like one another and share genetic material aren't necessarily interchangable.

It is therefore wholly inadequate to assert that a de-extinguished species will merely resume its former roles, and not cause problems. Furthermore, research on biological invasions shows that it is very difficult to accurately predict the abundance and impacts of newly introduced species. Consequently, we can expect some predictions about the effects of de-extinctions to be wrong, so that some de-extinctions anticipated to be benign will cause harm. It is therefore important that a plan for controlling or repairing damage be in place before these new organisms are released. We routinely assess the likely impacts of oil wells, and require that they be built and operated responsibly, but also require spill-response plans, because we know that some spills will occur despite our best efforts. De-extinguishing species will be far less certain than drilling and operating oil wells, so "spill response" plans will be essential.

Again, the usual response given to this concern is naïve and unsatisfactory: "we removed the species before, and if it becomes a problem, we can simply remove it again." Recall how we removed the passenger pigeon the first time: by felling millions of acres of forests and slaughtering countless birds for market. Does anyone really think that society would allow immense tracts of forest to be cut and millions of birds to be killed (for a market that doesn't even exist today) if passenger pigeon v.2.0 turned out to cause problems? Today's (and tomorrow's) world is vastly different from the world from which these species were removed, so the mechanism of their original extinction probably won't be available as a control method.

Instead of the glib answer that "we did it before, so we can do it again," we need a credible plan to remove problematic de-extinguished species or manage their impacts. Who will decide whether control or eradication is necessary? At what point in the de-extinction process will this decision be made? What tools or methods will be effective in controlling the species or its problems? And who will pay for these efforts? We know from experience with invasive species that control or eradication of nuisance species can be costly and difficult (or impossible), so developing such "spill" plans will be challenging. However, they will be as indispensible for de-extinction as for oil drilling.

Finally, we should ask why de-extinction needs to be done as soon as possible, and not deferred. It is natural that we are eager to bring species back from the dead as soon as we can. This eagerness generates nearly irresistible momentum, but we should resist this momentum and deliberately choose the best time (if ever) to pursue de-extinction. This may mean waiting until we gather information needed to assess the benefits and risks of releasing these new organisms into nature and develop a control plan.

The recent debate about whether to allow fracking in New York is instructive. This new technology can provide large benefits (formerly inaccessible natural gas), but rushing into fracking led to large environmental problems. One approach is to defer fracking. There is no hurry in getting the gas out of the ground (it will still be there tomorrow!), and we can expect to develop better technologies and environmental controls if we wait a bit. Not "no fracking ever," but "no fracking today."

A similar argument could be applied to de-extinction. There is no urgency to most of the cases that are being discussed, apart from the personal desires of some people; no greater difficulty in bringing back a species in 2100 rather than 2030. On the other hand, rushing headlong into de-extinction exposes us to unnecessary risks just as rushing headlong into fracking exposed us to unnecessary environmental damages. So we deserve a good answer to the question not only of why we should bring back the passenger pigeon, but why we should bring it back today.

As an invasion biologist, it's hard not to hear echoes of old enthusiasms in the arguments for de-extinction. ("The introduction of a few rabbits could do little harm and might provide a touch of home…[to Australia],"[1] "but that so fine a plant as this [water-chestnut], with its handsome leafy rosettes, and edible nuts, … can ever become a nuisance, I can scarcely believe."[2]) Over and over, naïve proponents of introductions seduced us with stories about how new species would improve ecosystems and benefit humans in myriad ways, their enthusiasm unchecked by any rigorous assessment of possible impacts or control plans.

Some of these introductions did bring benefits (although rarely the full benefits that were promised), but many caused large, lasting ecological and economic problems. This bitter experience should have taught us to be wary of the alluring stories now being told about de-extinction. If de-extinction is to proceed, we need serious consideration of its ecological effects, not romantic appeals to the imagination. Let's not repeat old mistakes with new species, no matter how technologically advanced their pedigrees.

Notes

1. Thomas Austin, 1859. Wikipedia.
2. George E. Davenport, Bulletin of the Torrey Botanical Club, Vol. 6, page 352.

Viewpoint 4

> *"In the more distant future, some scientists think we might be able to go further, genetically modifying animals to become better suited to their rapidly changing environments."*

Genetic Rescue Could Provide a Crucial Stop-Gap for Threatened Species

Laura Poppick

In the following viewpoint, Laura Poppick argues that, while genetic rescue is a promising technique that could possibly help many vulnerable species, it is not a panacea. It also is not without its problems, and scientists will need to tread lightly. Laura Poppick is a freelance journalist who writes about science, technology, and the environment for Smithsonian Magazine, Scientific American, *and* National Geographic, *among other publications.*

As you read, consider the following questions:

1. Why are pink pigeons susceptible to the parasite that is killing off its population?
2. What is outbreeding depression?
3. Why is the northern white rhino a "perfect candidate" for stem cell techniques, according to the viewpoint?

Like the doomed passenger pigeon in 1914, the pink pigeon of Mauritius is standing on the edge of a precipice. After watching all of its other pigeon cousins on this remote island go extinct—including the dodo, its infamous island-mate last seen in 1662—this rosy-hued bird is now looking down the dark gullet of extinction itself.

After yo-yo'ing down to a population of just around nine individuals in the 1990s, the studly birds are back up to a population of about 400 today. But that number is still small enough to leave them dangerously vulnerable. The pink pigeon's lack of genetic diversity has left it increasingly susceptible to a parasite-causing disease called trichomonosis, which kills more than half of its chicks and limits population growth.

Fortunately, it isn't 1662 anymore. Today, an evolving conservation tool could help pull these birds back from the brink of extinction: genetic rescue. It works by adding genetic diversity to these kinds of precariously numbered populations—by introducing specific individuals or, potentially, by someday directly editing their genes. If it works, this pigeon's future may once again be as rosy as its plumage.

"We want to try to give them the tools to fight this disease," says Camilla Ryan, a graduate student who studies the Mauritius pigeon with genomics researcher Matt Clark at England's Earlham University. "The birds don't have the numbers or potentially the genetic diversity to deal with the disease themselves."

Clark and Ryan are hoping to pull this population back on its feet by pinpointing the genes that make these birds so vulnerable to in the first place. Then, they'll sample captive pink pigeons in zoos and parks around the world in search of genes better suited to fight the disease, with the ultimate goal of potentially mating these with the wild population. The team has already generated genetic data from 180 different pink pigeons.

Still, the pair remain cautious in implementing a technique that has brewed controversy ever since it started becoming more readily implemented in the 1990s, in hallmark cases of rescuing

Florida panthers and Illinois prairie chickens. They aren't alone: Many conservationists argue that the approach could create unforeseen problems for species at risk, and that it doesn't resolve the underlying problems that push so many species to the brink of extinction, including habitat loss due to human development.

But as humans continue to encroach on wild habitats and alter global climate patterns, the situation for many species has become more dire. Now, many researchers are turning to genetic rescue as a viable tool to pull these most vulnerable species from the brink of extinction. In the more distant future, some scientists think we might be able to go further, genetically modifying animals to become better suited to their rapidly changing environments.

But let's not get too ahead of ourselves. For now, scientists are focused on sharpening their genomics tools.

When populations like the pink pigeon's shrink down to the double or even single digits, they experience something called inbreeding depression. Essentially, that means they have less diversity in their gene pool, which makes it harder for them to beat challenges in their environment. Signs of this have been found in numerous species, including an isolated population of wolves in Michigan where individuals started to develop an unusual arched posture and stubby tails—possible indicators of poor health.

Now, Ryan and Clark are scouring historic tissue samples from five museums across Europe to look for genes that older pink pigeons may have once had to fight off disease before inbreeding depression took hold. The team will then look for captive birds that may have maintained these historic helpful genes to mate them with the wild population.

Sounds fairly straightforward, right? Unfortunately, playing a genetic deity isn't that simple.

Each genotype you introduce into the existing population comes with its own pros and cons. So the team must be careful not to introduce new problems into the wild birds' immune systems, says Clark. "You could end up breeding a population that is very successful at fighting off Trichomonas, but what you have done is accidentally decreased the amount of diversity in the immune system," says Clark.

If that's the case, he adds, a new disease that they weren't prepared for could theoretically hit and wipe out the entire population.

Mating captive birds with wild birds also runs the risk of introducing genes that the captive birds had evolved to survive in captivity, weakening the wild bird's ability to survive in the wild. "By trying to help them out, you've made it worse," Clark says. This threat, called outbreeding depression, raises hackles amongst conservation biologists and is a primary argument against using genetic rescue more widely.

Yet despite these risks, several success stories have shown that genetic rescue can work. One of the major success stories conservationists point to is the Florida panther.

This large, iconic cat once lurked through the southeastern U.S in large numbers, enjoying its status as top predator and vital member of the ecosystem. But by the 1970s, habitat loss and hunting had shrunk the population to between 12 and 20 adults. Not only were their numbers dismal, but almost all of the male panthers showed signs of inbreeding depression, including undescended testicles, kinked tails and low sperm counts.

Conservationists didn't want to see this cat—which helped keep populations of white-tailed deer, wild hog, and other prey animals in check—go extinct. So in 1995, the U.S. Fish and Wildlife Service worked with a team of researchers to transfer eight female mountain lions from Texas to mate with the Florida panthers. They hoped the mountain lions, which are a subspecies of the panther, would revitalize the gene pool and boost the population size.

Stuart Pimm, a conservation ecologist at Duke University, says he had his doubts at first. If you were trying to rescue a species that had become so rare that it showed genetic damage, he believed, then it was already too late to save them. Many of his colleagues agreed. "You were treating the symptom rather than the cause," Pimm says, citing habitat loss as the major cause in this case.

But the researchers went ahead, and mated the panthers and the mountain lions. Amazingly, their efforts seemed to work. The panther population grew and the next generation appeared free of kinked tails, undescended testicles, and other signs of inbreeding. "All of those things disappeared," says Pimm. Ten years later, Pimm ran a follow-up study showing they had sustained a growing population free of these signs of inbreeding depression.

"It was fast, it was a very effective process," he says now.

Other success stories popped up in the 1990s. Great prairie chicken populations grew for the first time in decades (though more recent studies question the role of genetic rescue in this success), along with the Swedish adder, a venomous snake that had suffered from inbreeding. Today, Pimm has changed his tune: He now believes genetic rescue can be an excellent tool in a conservationist's toolbox, and is considering using it to protect other top predators, including lions in Africa.

As researchers around the world consider implementing genetic rescue, they must better understand how the risk of outbreeding depression could differ from species to species. Unfortunately, because genetic rescue has been so controversial, few cases exist that could offer this information.

Even the success stories of the panthers, chickens and adders hold limited information regarding how the mechanism might transfer from one species to another, says Andrew Whiteley, a conservation genomics researcher at the University of Montana. That's partly because these cases weren't done systematically—they were more of a last-ditch effort to save a critically endangered species.

"Those were done in response to a pressing management concern, they weren't really done to test the concept of genetic rescue in an experimentally rigorous way," says Whiteley. "So those uncertainties are going to remain."

Working to fill those knowledge gaps, Whitely has been conducting experiments with brook trout—a species easier to experimentally study than large predators—in which his team has moved fish into four different isolated populations and introduced fish from elsewhere to mate with them. Preliminary results suggest that the first round of matings were successful, but the real measure of success will come with the second generation's ability to survive and reproduce—this is where symptoms of outbreeding depression tend to arise.

He plans to conduct a comprehensive assessment of the second generation's ability to survive and reproduce, building a so-called pedigree to see how genes flow through the system. "And ultimately dig in with genomics to understand at the genome level what happened when this pulse of gene flow entered this small population," says Whiteley. "Those are the types of data we need to be able to make solid recommendations."

If the traditional form of genetic rescue is considered controversial, a newly developing iteration will like start a far louder hullabaloo. Today, biologists are considering literal tinkering with animal genomes, by genetically engineering them to have certain traits.

Robert Fleischer, head of the Center for Conservation Genomics at Smithsonian's National Zoo & Conservation Biology Institute, is considering this option to make birds in Hawaii resistant to or tolerant of avian malaria, a human-introduced pathogen devastating many Hawaiian bird populations today. But researchers in his group and elsewhere say they are just in the preliminary stages of investigating this technique.

"We are not at the stage of doing any rescuing yet, we are just setting the stage for doing that in the future if it will work out," says Fleischer.

Oliver Ryder, director of Conservation Genetics at San Diego Zoo Global, says these techniques could someday prove invaluable, but that broader discussions about the ethics and logistics would need to come first. Within those discussions, researchers would need to weigh the risks associated with each case—including the risk that the efforts simply wouldn't work.

"In spite of the efforts, the pathogen would find a way around the solution or the engineering," says Ryder, "so all of the effort would not be sufficient to keep the species from going extinct."

Ryder is involved in a broader effort to develop yet another genetic rescue approach, and is interested in using it to save the Northern White Rhino. The technique, which is still years away, would use stem cell technology to produce eggs and sperm from frozen Northern White Rhinos cells stored at the San Diego Zoo Global. His team is also looking into using frozen sperm to create embryos from eggs obtained either from the last living females or through stem cell techniques. They would then theoretically transfer embryos into closely related rhinos, who would serve as surrogates.

This rhino is the perfect candidate for such an approach, in part because there are only three of these individuals left that are all unable to breed naturally, Ryder says. "The Northern White Rhino is functionally extinct," says Ryder. "The only way to keep it from going extinct would be to genetically rescue it using advanced genetic and reproductive technologies."

For now, researchers generally agree that traditional genetic rescue without genetic modification offers the most immediate conservation solution. However, it will never be the end-all solution to saving degrading populations. Instead, it offers a stop-gap opportunity to deal other overlying issues like reducing isolation and improving habitat, says Chris Funk, a researcher at Colorado State University who has conducted studies on Trinidadian guppies to track when and how outbreeding depression may arise.

Funk, like Pimm, at first called himself a skeptic—not because he didn't believe genetic rescue could work, but because he considered himself a purist when it came to conservation. But as more and more populations become isolated and threatened by increasing human pressures and development, he says he has come to realize that some compromises may be necessary. "There is accumulating evidence that it can work in a lot of circumstances," says Funk.

"We are not going to have the luxury to have this purist attitude," he continues. "If we want these populations on the landscape, we are going to have to use genetic rescue to keep them from going extinct."

Viewpoint 5

> *"As the genetically 'tamed' organisms breed with wild ones, the CRISPR gene drive cuts the original version and replaces it with the edited one. Now, in the next generation, all the offspring are guaranteed to inherit it."*

Gene Drives Can Eliminate Invasive Species, but Researchers Must Proceed with Caution

Kathiann Kowalski

In the following viewpoint, Kathiann Kowalski explores a gene-editing tool called a gene drive. Used successfully (and ethically), it could result in the relatively rapid elimination of invasive species responsible for threatening animal and wildlife populations. The potential danger, the author notes, is in the wiping out of such species, which may be useful to certain other ecosystems. Kathiann Kowalski is a health and science writer and reporter.

As you read, consider the following questions:

1. What does an evolutionary ecologist study?
2. What is a gene drive?
3. What ethical questions arise when considering combining gene drives and CRISPR technology?

"Can DNA Editing Save Endangered Species?" by Kathiann Kowalski, Society for Science & the Public, March 6, 2018. Reprinted by permission.

Kiwis and other native birds in New Zealand are in trouble. In the 19th century, European traders and immigrants introduced many foreign rats, stoats and other animals to the South Pacific island nation. Since then, many of these non-native animals—known as invasive species—have been preying on the native birds, some of which don't fly. New Zealand's leaders want to get rid of the invaders. And a new technology could help. But scientists are now questioning whether that is a smart thing to do.

Kevin Esvelt is an evolutionary ecologist at the Massachusetts Institute of Technology in Cambridge. An evolutionary ecologist studies the genetics of living things and how species have changed over time. "You need to be very careful," Esvelt says. It's always possible, he notes, that some "solution" might cause problems elsewhere in an ecosystem.

Esvelt is talking with people in New Zealand about a plan. They're considering use of a type of gene-editing tool known as a gene drive. It can copy and paste itself into the genome of an organism. (A genome is the complete set of genetic instructions in an organism.) Once the gene drive is inside the genome, it could change the genes of some invasive species in a way that would make that species die off at sites where it doesn't belong.

That may sound like a good thing. Indeed, many scientists hope it will be. Still, they have concerns. After all, if a gene drive "escapes," it could kill that targeted species even in places where it does belong.

Tina Saey of *Science News* magazine has a doctorate degree in molecular genetics. She has covered gene editing and gene drives a lot. In an award-winning feature story in the magazine, she notes: "Researchers have designed ways to keep [gene drives] confined in the lab." However, she adds, "no such safety nets exist for gene drives released into the wild."

Wiping out an entire species, even if it's a pest, raises questions about whether such a move would be the right thing to do. To date, she points out, scientists and policymakers are only just starting to think about this.

How It Works

In recent years, a new and very popular tool has been available to tinker with genes. It's known as CRISPR/Cas9. Most people just call it CRISPR. (That's much shorter than using its entire name: "clustered regularly interspaced short palindromic repeats.") The Cas9 part is an enzyme. It's a molecular scissors, of sorts, that cuts DNA.

Scientists inject Cas9 into a cell in which they want to alter DNA. But Cas9 is blind and doesn't know where to make cuts. It needs a buddy, like a guide dog, to show it where to snip. In this case, the guide dog is a small piece of another type of genetic material, called RNA. The guide RNA shows Cas9 where to cut.

Guide RNAs are very picky. They will only take Cas9 to one particular place in the genome. It's similar to a guide dog leading its owner to one particular subway station and to the correct track. Even though there are many subway stations and multiple tracks, only one is the right one.

Once Cas9 and its guide reach their destination, the scissors snips the DNA. Then, other things can happen. One possibility is that the cell can repair the cut. Sometimes the repair is done by sticking the cut ends back together. That can break the gene. Sometimes the repair fixes a previously broken gene, by using a healthy copy of the gene as a pattern. Scientists have used this RNA-enzyme combo to break and fix genes in many types of animals.

Another possibility is that a piece of DNA that the researchers have injected into the cell (along with Cas9) can be pasted into the cut section. Scientists use this method to insert genes into plants and animals at precise locations.

Gene drives take the CRISPR system a step further.

A gene drive uses an extra piece of DNA to paste into the cut. That extra DNA contains the code to make the CRISPR system again. It's like a combination scissors and copy machine that can make copies of itself.

When an animal or plant carrying a gene drive mates, its eggs or sperm will make the scissors protein and the guide RNA. When the egg or sperm from the organism with the gene drive fuses to an egg or sperm from an unaltered organism, the gene drive goes to work. Cas9 cuts the unaltered DNA in the place where the guide RNA shows it to. Then, the cell repairs the break by putting in a copy of the gene drive. It's that extra copying step that makes a gene drive different from regular CRISPR.

What Makes a Gene Drive Special

Normally a parent has a 50/50 chance of passing any given gene along to its offspring. But gene drives take over any unaltered version of the target gene. So, they can be passed along almost 100 percent of the time. That's why they are called gene drives—because they break the 50/50 genetic speed limit.

Scientists have used gene drives in the lab to alter eye color in fruit flies. They have tinkered with yeast. Two separate groups have made CRISPR gene drives to stop mosquitoes from transmitting malaria. (One group of researchers altered the mosquitoes so that the insects can't carry the malaria parasite. The other group altered genes so that the mosquitoes can no longer reproduce.)

CRISPR gene drives could set the stage to make gene edits in nearly every member of a selected species. How? Scientists add the new gene they want to alter—let's call it a "taming" one—to the targeted species. Then the CRISPR gene drive makes this change whenever it finds a wild (untweaked) version of the gene.

As the genetically "tamed" organisms breed with wild ones, the CRISPR gene drive "cuts the original version and replaces it with the edited one," Esvelt explains. Now, "in the next generation, all the offspring are guaranteed to inherit it. And again. And again. And again." Eventually, practically every organism in a population will be born with the newly inserted taming gene.

Breaking That Speed Limit

In a small population, that change can take just 12 to 24 generations. For short-lived animals like a rat, that may amount to only several years. If any organisms with the altered gene go elsewhere, they can spread that gene drive into a new population. For instance, Esvelt notes, "Rats are really good stowaways [on ships]." Or people could intentionally move them. Just a handful of altered organisms released into a new population should be able to quickly spread the gene drive through all of them, Esvelt says.

He even suggests a humane way to kill off a rat population that threatened local bird species: Add a gene that makes the rats infertile. Individual rats wouldn't suffer. But they couldn't have more babies. Over time, the local population would die out. And the rats' threat to the birds would go away.

But even rats have native populations where an ecosystem depends on them. So scientists don't want to kill them off everywhere in the world. Otherwise, that could throw off the ecological balance somewhere else. Esvelt's group has proposed a way to limit that risk.

"We call this a daisy drive, because it involves creating a gene-drive daisy chain," he explains. Just as each flower in a chain of daisies is a separate unit, each part of the "daisy" gene drive would have part of the instructions for CRISPR and the gene drive. And those parts are scattered around in different places in the genome. Because only half of a parent's DNA is passed on to offspring, some of the pieces won't get inherited in the next generation. Without all of the pieces in one organism, the gene drive eventually gets a flat tire and can't drive anymore.

Esvelt has gotten the daisy chain gene drive to work in the lab with tiny worms known as nematodes. The results are "very preliminary," he says. However, he believes, it's time to start talking about the idea.

Do We Have the Right?

Todd Kuiken is an environmental scientist at North Carolina State University in Raleigh. He and Esvelt talked about gene drives and CRISPR on October 6. They were taking part in the Society of Environmental Journalists' annual meeting in Pittsburgh, Pa. Kuiken agrees that lots of people should think hard and talk about whether and how to couple gene drives and CRISPR.

"Do we as humans really have the right to do this?" Kuiken asks. That's a big question. What he means is that there's a lot at stake with a version of a gene drive that is designed to spread a change in the environment forever. Even with the daisy chain, he wonders whether humans have the right "to remove one species from one area where we don't want it, or that we don't think is good for it."

Also, he asks, "where do you field-test a gene drive?" After all, the animals people want to change don't stay put. They tend to roam about an ecosystem.

No one has clear answers on what is the right thing to do. Nor is it clear who should have the right to make the final call, Kuiken says. Yet that doesn't mean the technology shouldn't be used at all, he adds. Indeed, he noted, if people wait too long, it may be too late to save an endangered species.

Periodical and Internet Sources Bibliography

The following articles have been selected to supplement the diverse views presented in this chapter.

Justine Calma, "Don't Count on Resurrected Woolly Mammoths to Combat Climate Change," The Verge, September 15, 2021, https://www.theverge.com/2021/9/15/22673392/woolly-mammoth-de-extinction-colossal-biodiversity-climate-change.

Paul Ehrlich and Anne H. Ehrlich, "A Case Against De-Extinction: It's a Fascinating, but Dumb Idea," *Yale Environment 360*, January 13, 2014, https://e360.yale.edu/features/the_case_against_de-extinction_its_a_fascinating_but_dumb_idea.

Sherryn Groch, "'The De-Extinction Club': Could We Resurrect Mammoths, Tassie Tigers, and Dinosaurs?" *Sydney Morning Herald*, July 25, 2021, https://www.smh.com.au/national/the-de-extinction-club-could-we-resurrect-mammoths-tassie-tigers-and-dinosaurs-20210703-p586jg.html.

Julian Koplin and Christopher Gyngell, "Bringing Woolly Mammoths Back from Extinction Might Not Be Such a Bad Idea—Ethicists Explain," The Conversation, September 15, 2012, https://theconversation.com/bringing-woolly-mammoths-back-from-extinction-might-not-be-such-a-bad-idea-ethicists-explain-167892.

Amy Dockser Marcus, "Meet the Scientists Bringing Extinct Species Back from the Dead," *Wall Street Journal*, October 11, 2018, https://www.wsj.com/articles/meet-the-scientists-bringing-extinct-species-back-from-the-dead-1539093600.

Helen Pilcher, "Can We Bring Extinct Animals Back from the Dead?" *Science Focus*, July 10, 2020, https://www.sciencefocus.com/nature/de-extinction-can-we-bring-extinct-animals-back-from-the-dead/.

W. S. Roberts, "The Booming Call of De-Extinction," *The Scientist*, October 19, 2020, https://www.the-scientist.com/news-opinion/the-booming-call-of-de-extinction-68057.

David Shultz, "Bringing Extinct Species Back from the Dead Could Hurt—Not Help—Conservation Efforts," *Science*, February 27,

2017, https://www.science.org/content/article/bringing-extinct-species-back-dead-could-hurt-not-help-conservation-efforts.

Vir Singh, "The Jury Is Still Out on the De-Extinction of the Woolly Mammoth," Down to Earth, October 19, 2021, https://www.downtoearth.org.in/blog/wildlife-biodiversity/the-jury-is-still-out-on-the-de-extinction-of-the-woolly-mammoth-79748.

Carl Zimmer, "A New Company with a Wild Mission: Bring Back the Woolly Mammoth," *New York Times*, September 13, 2021, https://www.nytimes.com/2021/09/13/science/colossal-woolly-mammoth-DNA.html.

OPPOSING VIEWPOINTS® SERIES

Chapter 4

Should Genetically Modified Foods Be a Part of Our Food System?

Chapter Preface

Genetically modified foods were a part of the public conversation long before CRISPR was developed. However, new technologies for adapting foods for animals as well as for people have brought the topic back to the public's attention. Most of the questions are the same as they have been for years: Are GMO foods safe for human consumption? Are GMO crops safe for the environment? Do GMO crops reduce the need for pesticides, or do they increase the need? Should products containing GMOs be labeled as such?

Most of the viewpoints in this chapter address one or the other of these issues. However, in the last decade, there has been a new use for genetic engineering that affects the food system, though not so much those who eat as those who are eaten (or provide products, such as eggs and milk, that are eaten).

Most people acknowledge that animals on factory farms suffer a great deal. Long before they are slaughtered, farm animals are subject to conditions like being crammed in small cages, crowded into feedlots, having body parts removed (such as beaks and wings and horns), and many more routine cruelties. Even those people who believe this is necessary to provide enough food for humans would like to find a solution that decreases suffering for animals. One proposed solution is to use genetic engineering to remove the animals' ability to experience pain. This is called "disenhancement."

The viewpoints that follow tackle the complex debates surrounding GMO foods.

Viewpoint 1

> *"Although GMOs are in a lot of the foods we eat, most of the GMO crops grown in the United States are used for animal food."*

According to the FDA, Our Foods, GMO and Otherwise, Are Safe

USFDA

In the following viewpoint, the US Food and Drug Administration (FDA) argues that most of us are probably eating genetically modified (GMO) foods. This is not because most foods are GMO, but because the ones that are GMO are among the most commonly grown crops and are used as ingredients in other foods as well as being foods in their own right. However, most GMO crops are fed to animals. In addition, some medicines and many textiles are made from GMO plants. The FDA assures us, however, that this GMO food is safe and labeled in accordance with federal law. The US Food and Drug Administration is responsible for protecting the public's health by ensuring the safety of the nation's food supply, among other things.

As you read, consider the following questions:

1. What are most GMO food products used for, according to the viewpoint?
2. What are soybeans typically used for?
3. Why are animals that feed on GMO foods not themselves GMO when they are eaten?

"GMO Crops, Animal Food, and Beyond," US Food and Drug Administration, September 28, 2020.

It is very likely you are eating foods and food products that are made with ingredients that come from GMO crops. Many GMO crops are used to make ingredients that Americans eat, such as cornstarch, corn syrup, corn oil, soybean oil, canola oil, or granulated sugar. A few fresh fruits and vegetables are available in GMO varieties, including potatoes, summer squash, apples, and papayas. Although GMOs are in a lot of the foods we eat, most of the GMO crops grown in the United States are used for animal food.

To make it easier for consumers to know if the foods they eat contain GMO ingredients, the U.S. Department of Agriculture maintains a list of bioengineered foods available throughout the world. Additionally, you will start seeing the "bioengineered" label on some of the foods we eat because of the new National Bioengineered Food Disclosure Standard.

What GMO Crops Are Grown and Sold in the United States?

Only a few types of GMO crops are grown in the United States, but some of these GMOs make up a large percentage of the crop grown (e.g., soybeans, corn, sugar beets, canola, and cotton).

In 2018, GMO soybeans made up 94% of all soybeans planted, GMO cotton made up 94% of all cotton planted, and 92% of corn planted was GMO corn.

In 2013, GMO canola made up 95% of canola planted while GMO sugar beets made up 99.9% of all sugar beets harvested.

Most GMO plants are used to make ingredients that are then used in other food products, for example, cornstarch made from GMO corn or sugar made from GMO sugar beets.

Corn

Corn is the most commonly grown crop in the United States, and most of it is GMO. Most GMO corn is created to resist insect pests or tolerate herbicides. *Bacillus thuringiensis* (Bt) corn is a GMO corn that produces proteins that are toxic to certain insect pests but not to humans, pets, livestock, or other animals. These are the same types of proteins that organic farmers use to control insect pests, and they do not harm other, beneficial insects such as ladybugs. GMO Bt corn reduces the need for spraying insecticides while still preventing insect damage. While a lot of GMO corn goes into processed foods and drinks, most of it is used to feed livestock, like cows, and poultry, like chickens.

Soybean

Most soy grown in the United States is GMO soy. Most GMO soy is used for food for animals, predominantly poultry and livestock, and making soybean oil. It is also used as ingredients (lecithin, emulsifiers, and proteins) in processed foods.

Cotton

GMO cotton was created to be resistant to bollworms and helped revive the Alabama cotton industry. GMO cotton not only provides a reliable source of cotton for the textile industry, it is also used to make cottonseed oil, which is used in packaged foods and in many restaurants for frying. GMO cottonseed meal and hulls are also used in food for animals.

Potato

Some GMO potatoes were developed to resist insect pests and disease. In addition, some GMO potato varieties have been developed to resist bruising and browning that can occur when potatoes are packaged, stored, and transported, or even cut in your kitchen. While browning does not change the quality of the potato, it often leads to food being unnecessarily thrown away because people mistakenly believe browned food is spoiled.

Papaya

By the 1990s, ringspot virus disease had nearly wiped out Hawaii's papaya crop, and in the process almost destroyed the papaya industry in Hawaii. A GMO papaya, named the Rainbow papaya, was created to resist ringspot virus. This GMO saved papaya farming on the Hawaiian Islands.

Summer Squash

GMO summer squash is resistant to some plant viruses. Squash was one of the first GMOs on the market, but it is not widely grown.

Canola

GMO canola is used mostly to make cooking oil and margarine. Canola seed meal can also be used in food for animals. Canola oil is used in many packaged foods to improve food consistency. Most GMO canola is resistant to herbicides and helps farmers to more easily control weeds in their fields.

Alfalfa

GMO alfalfa is primarily used to feed cattle—mostly dairy cows. Most GMO alfalfa is resistant to herbicides, allowing farmers to spray the crops to protect them against destructive weeds that can reduce alfalfa production and lower the nutritional quality of the hay.

Apple

A few varieties of GMO apples were developed to resist browning after being cut. This helps cut down on food waste, as many consumers think brown apples are spoiled.

Sugar Beet

Sugar beets are used to make granulated sugar. More than half the granulated sugar packaged for grocery store shelves is made from GMO sugar beets. Because GMO sugar beets are resistant to herbicides, growing GMO sugar beets helps farmers control weeds in their fields.

What About Animals That Eat Food Made from GMO Crops?

More than 95% of animals used for meat and dairy in the United States eat GMO crops. Independent studies show that there is no difference in how GMO and non-GMO foods affect the health and safety of animals. The DNA in the GMO food does not transfer to the animal that eats it. This means that animals that eat GMO food do not turn into GMOs. If it did, an animal would have the DNA of any food it ate, GMO or not. In other words, cows do not become the grass they eat and chickens don't become the corn they eat.

Similarly, the DNA from GMO animal food does not make it into the meat, eggs, or milk from the animal. Research shows that foods like eggs, dairy products, and meat that come from animals that eat GMO food are equal in nutritional value, safety, and quality to foods made from animals that eat only non-GMO food.

Who Makes Sure Animal Food Is Safe?

The U.S. Food and Drug Administration (FDA) is the primary regulatory agency responsible for ensuring the safety of GMO and non-GMO food for animals. The FDA Center for Veterinary Medicine manages this responsibility. FDA requires that all food for animals, like food for human foods, be safe for animals to eat, be produced under clean conditions, contain no harmful substances, and be accurately labeled.

Are There GMO Animals in the Food Supply?

There soon will be. FDA has approved an application that allows the marketing of the AquAdvantage Salmon, an Atlantic salmon that has been genetically modified to reach an important growth point faster. FDA determined that AquAdvantage Salmon is as safe to eat and as nutritious as non-GMO Atlantic salmon. FDA also found that its approval of the application for this salmon would not significantly impact the U.S. environment.

Are GMOs Used to Make Anything Besides Food?

When you hear the term "GMO" you probably think of food. However, techniques used to create GMOs are important in creating some medicines as well. In fact, genetic engineering, which is the process used to create GMOs, was first used to make human insulin, a medicine used to treat diabetes. Medicines developed through genetic engineering go through an in-depth FDA approval process. All medicines must be proven to be safe and effective before they are approved for human use. GMOs are also used in the textile industry. Some GMO cotton plants are used to create cotton fiber that is then used to make fabric for clothing and other materials.

Viewpoint 2

> *"Scientists can't predict with absolute certainty what would happen in the event of an escape. The real world is just too complicated."*

GMO Salmon Is Only Safe If It Doesn't Get Out

Jessie Rack

In the following viewpoint, Jessie Rack argues that for all their benefits, GMO foods pose the risk of tampering with natural ecosystems. At the time of this writing, most genetically modified foods were plant based. However, one company, AquaBounty Technologies, was working to get approval for a salmon that was modified to grow much faster than ordinary farm-raised fish. The problem, critics argued, wasn't with the fish itself, but with the harm it might do to wild salmon populations should it escape from hatcheries. Three years after this viewpoint was written, the US Food and Drug Administration approved AquaBounty's GMO salmon for sale in the United States. Jessie Rack is an ecologist, educator, and science writer.

As you read, consider the following questions:

1. Why was it taking so long for AquaBounty to get its GMO salmon approved?
2. How did altering one gene in salmon affect other traits?
3. What is the risk to wild salmon?

While the debate over whether to label foods containing GMO ingredients plays out across the country, another engineered food has long been waiting to hit grocery stores: genetically modified salmon.

Produced by Massachusetts-based biotech firm AquaBounty Technologies, the fish is an Atlantic salmon engineered to grow twice as fast as its conventional, farm-raised counterpart. But AquaBounty's fish has been languishing in the regulatory process: The company has been trying to get the U.S. Food and Drug Administration to approve its salmon for sale for nearly 20 years.

One concern repeatedly raised by critics who don't want the FDA to give the transgenic fish the green light: What would happen if these fish got out of the land-based facilities where they're grown and escaped into the wild? Would genetically modified salmon push out their wild counterparts or permanently alter habitat? In a review paper published this month in the journal *BioScience*, scientists tackle that very question.

Robert H. Devlin, a scientist at Fisheries and Oceans Canada, led a team that reviewed more than 80 studies analyzing growth, behavior and other trait differences between genetically modified and unaltered fish. The scientists used this to predict what might happen if fish with modified traits were unleashed in nature.

Genetically modified salmon contain the growth hormone gene from one fish, combined with the promoter of an antifreeze gene from another. This combination both increases and speeds up growth, so the salmon grow faster.

Altering a fish's genes also changes other traits, the review found. Genetically modified salmon eat more food, spend more time near the surface of the water, and don't tend to associate in groups. They develop at a dramatically faster rate, and their immune function is reduced.

But would these altered traits help genetically modified salmon outcompete wild salmon, while at the same time making them less likely to thrive in nature? It's unclear, says Fredrik Sundström, one of the study authors and an ecologist at Uppsala University in Sweden. He stresses that we can't assume genetically modified fish would perish quickly in nature, just because they didn't evolve there.

It's analogous, he says, to invasive species. "Invasive species also didn't evolve in the environment where they are now invading, and they still are able to survive and flourish. We could argue along the same lines with the [genetically modified] fish."

Are Genetically Modified Organisms Safe?

Because GMOs have modifications that do not occur naturally, governments believe it is important to assess their potential effects on human health and on the environment.

For this, regulations have been established in order to keep under control the production, assessment and commercialization of GMOs; and the WHO together with the Food and Agriculture Organization (FAO), have developed documents regarding GMOs risk assessment.

According to this and to other regulations, GMOs are evaluated to determine their potential toxicity towards the human being and the environment, their potential to cause allergies, their components and their nutritional and toxic characteristics, how stable the gene that was introduced is and any side effects that the introduction of this gene might have.

GMOs that are currently available in the market went through all the required assessments in order for them to be suitable for human consumption.

Despite obvious differences between genetically engineered and wild salmon, predicting what could happen in a real escape is challenging. According to Sundström, "it's very difficult to predict any ecological consequences before these fish are actually in nature, when it's kind of too late to do anything about it."

But how likely is an escape, really?

"Virtually impossible," says Dave Conley, director of corporate communications for AquaBounty. "We have in essence mitigated all the possible risk scenarios by combining biological and physical methods to reduce those risks to essentially zero," he tells The Salt via email.

AquaBounty grows its salmon in tanks on land, rather than in open-ocean tanks. According to the FDA's environmental

So, yes, they are safe, and they continue under evaluation, now that they are consumed, in order to ensure that they are safe on a long-term basis.

Despite of the regulations that exist to ensure the safety of GMOs, a large number of individuals and non-governmental organizations have raised concerns regarding the safety of these products towards human health and the environment.

Why? Because the genetic modification of a plant or any other organism may result in the alteration of the genetics of the consumer and of similar organismal species, causing disruption in the environment and the promotion of certain diseases related to genetic alteration, not only in humans but also in other beings, such as wild plants, insects and other animals.

Concerns also relate to the fact that companies will claim ownership on the GMOs that they develop, monopolizing the production of these products and introducing monocultures, which would threaten to reduce the variety of products that can be grown in a certain region. These could potentially harm local agricultural practices and increase the price of GMO products that would be offered to the general public.

"Genetically Modified Organisms: Are They Dangerous?" by Irina Vazquez, SteadyHealth, August 27, 2014.

assessment of AquaBounty's fish, an additional combination of screens, filters and netting block access to drains and pipes that might provide means of escape.

What's more, AquaBounty says its salmon will be all-female and sterile, so if they do escape, they will fail to reproduce.

But critics remain unswayed by such assurances. Environmentalists question just how dependable the company's containment methods are.

As Dana Perls of the environmental group Friends of the Earth points out, "Land-based doesn't mean not near a river." A fish egg production facility on Prince Edward Island is located next to an estuary, while another facility in Panama, where the fish are allowed to mature, is close to a river, according to the FDA documents. She calls escapes "an unavoidable consequence" of fish farming.

There are also questions about the process used to render the fish sterile. It carries a very small rate of failure, but if a large number of fish escaped at once, a few fertile fish could introduce the transgenes into the wild population.

Sundström attests that the risk of escape is, for the most part, in the future. "We are expecting very little risk at the moment, because there are very few facilities that actually hold these fish. I think what's a worry to some people is if it becomes commercialized and you find these kind of fish in millions of hatcheries around the world."

If that were to happen, he says, the concern is that growers might become lax about containment methods, and then it would just be a matter of time before a fish—or a few—got out.

Sundström says scientists can't predict with absolute certainty what would happen in the event of an escape. The real world is just too complicated. "You have to accept a certain amount of risk," he says.

And how much risk is too much? "It's not my thing to answer." He says that's for regulators to decide.

VIEWPOINT 3

> *"Ideally we'd be able to increase food access in ways that don't include risk, but there are few, if any, options at this level of potential positive impact that are risk-free."*

Gene Modification of Crops Can Reduce Hunger Around the Globe

Utibe Effiong and Ramadhani Noor

In the following viewpoint, Utibe Effiong and Ramadhani Noor argue that GM crops can be the solution to the world's hunger crisis. But the authors caution that the potential risks and ethical quandaries involved in creating GM foods necessitate a careful framework of government regulations. Utibe Effiong is resident physician at St. Mary Mercy Hospital and research scientist for the Exposure Research Laboratory at the University of Michigan. Ramadhani Noor is a doctor of science in nutrition epidemiology and consultant at the World Bank.

"Can Gene Editing Provide a Solution to Global Hunger?" by Utibe Effiong and Ramadhani Noor, The Conversation, July 6, 2015. https://theconversation.com/can-gene-editing-provide-a-solution-to-global-hunger-43444.

As you read, consider the following questions:

1. How many people on Earth don't have enough food?
2. Why did scientists alter the genes of potatoes?
3. Why do the authors suggest that the USDA look to the EU when regulating GMO crops?

According to the World Food Program, some 795 million people—one in nine people on earth—don't have enough food to lead a healthy active life. That will only get worse with the next global food crisis, predicted to occur within four years by experts at the recent Third International Conference on Global Warming and Food Security.

Unprecedented population growth, increasing conflict and displacement, natural calamities and emergence of major epidemics are some of the factors that will compound complexities of global food security over the coming years. And recent natural disasters in food-exporting Asian and African countries, as well as regions like California, may hasten a crisis.

In the face of these facts, any technique that can improve food production would be a welcome development. To counteract the coming problem, it is imperative to try novel and daring solutions across the agricultural food chain, including the gene modification of crops. While genetically modified (GM) crops could be our best hope for feeding an increasingly hungry planet, they need to be developed within a regulatory framework that takes potential risks into account and protects farmers, consumers and the environment.

GM Crops in the Developing World

Gene modification can produce nutrient-rich, highly productive, drought- and pest-resistant crop varieties much needed by small-scale farmers globally. For example, scientists at biotech company Cellectis have extended the shelf life of potatoes by disabling a single gene that promotes accumulation of sweet sugars within the tuber. Using this technique, they also reduced its production of cancer-promoting agents including acrylamide, which is often produced when a potato is fried.

One can imagine these kinds of improvements being of particular interest to farmers in Africa and the rest of the developing world, who rely on staple crops including corn, rice, potatoes and soy. Along with genetically modified cotton, GM corn and soy are currently grown in the African countries of Burkina Faso, Egypt and South Africa.

In most African countries, however, GM crops remain a farfetched idea. Despite important economic progress and agricultural successes, according to the Food and Agriculture Organization, Africa remains the world's most food-insecure continent. One-third of our continent's population is chronically undernourished. Chronic malnutrition, or "hidden hunger," though often invisible, is devastating and deadly. Over half of children's deaths globally can be averted if children have access to nutritious foods.

How Does Gene Editing Work?

Conventionally, the production of genetically modified organisms involves inserting desired foreign genes into the genome of a plant or animal. But a different technique known as gene editing modifies plant, as well as animal and human, genomes without the introduction of foreign genetic materials.

Gene editing uses biological catalysts called transcription activator-like effector nucleases (TALENs) that can be engineered to bind to any DNA sequence. Scientists can introduce these enzymes into living cells where they cut out unwanted pieces of DNA, in effect editing the genome. This technique, known as TALEN mediated genome engineering, is also referred to as Genome Editing with Engineered Nucleases.

Genome editing is not a new idea. It has been used to create gene edits in human stem cells as well as in worms, fish, mice and cattle with varying degrees of success. In the laboratory, TALENs have also been used to successfully correct the genetic error underlying diseases such as sickle cell anemia.

In crop science, gene editing has been used to make Cellectis's less sugary potato, as well as a soybean containing high levels of omega-3. The first commercial application of this technology in a plant for human consumption was approved this spring, when the US company Cibus announced an edited version of canola. The new canola plant is designed to grow well even when farmers apply particular herbicides that are used to control glyphosate-resistant weeds. Now there is talk of using this technique to manipulate photosynthesis to produce more food. Researchers at the International Rice Research Institute in the Philippines have engineered rice plants to extract energy from sunlight far more efficiently than they do now.

Risks Along with the Promise

Techniques for genetic engineering are not perfect. Significant genetic errors have been produced by the commonly applied techniques of genome editing, including TALENs, in the past. In laboratory models, off-target events that produce unwanted mutations, sometimes with fatal results, have been described in plants, fish and human cells.

For now, there remain many uncertainties about the impact of gene-edited organisms on the environment and health. While gene editing may not introduce foreign genetic material, the technology definitely changes the composition of the product at a very fundamental level. Research is currently under way to improve these techniques, reduce the frequency of unwanted mutations and improve the safety of genome editing.

While GMO crops cover 170 million hectares of land globally, representing 11% of all arable land, they remain controversial. Golden rice, for example, promises to save one million children a year from vitamin A-related mortality. Despite biotech company

Sygenta offering the license to grow golden rice free of charge for humanitarian use, its approval has been stalled in most settings.

Of course, ideally we'd be able to increase food access in ways that don't include risk, but there are few, if any, options at this level of potential positive impact that are risk-free.

Regulatory Protections

Because strict regulatory oversight is mostly lacking on GM techniques including genome editing, it's conceivable that biotech companies may develop experimental gene-edited crops for testing in developing countries where the need for food is greater than the political will to protect the masses.

India's experience with GMO crops makes the point. The country poorly regulated adoption of genetic engineering. While still a multifarious issue, activists contend that indeptedness and crop failure—both, they say, inevitable outcomes of the corporate model of industrial agriculture introduced in India—have further stressed some Indian farmers.

Interestingly, the move toward genome editing as the favored approach to genetic engineering may, at least in part, provide some leeway for biotech companies to avoid regulation. Genome editing using TALENs and similar techniques are either outside the jurisdiction of the US Department of Agriculture or were not envisioned when existing regulations were created.

The USDA currently relies on a product-based regulatory framework that focuses less on the technology used to develop the crop and more on the inherent risk of the final product. The emphasis is on any potential risk the new traits or attributes introduced into the plant pose to the public or the environment. But considering the reality of unanticipated, and often controversial, novel techniques of food production, it might be a better idea for the USDA to utilize process-based regulations as done by the EU, Argentina, Brazil, and several other countries. In those countries, the regulators focus on how food crops are developed, not just on the final outcome.

The world needs more nutrient-rich, environmentally friendly food production. More gene editing in food crops makes sense, but only with prudent regulatory mechanisms in place to ensure the safety of these new approaches to food availability. We don't want to see more harm than good done as we seek to address the issue of global food security.

Viewpoint 4

> *"We are using genome editing technologies to introduce new plant traits by directly rewriting the plants' genetic code."*

CRISPR-Modified Crops Don't Count as GMOs

Yi Li

In the following viewpoint, Yi Li argues that CRISPR technology has been used successfully to engineer plants with the intention of boosting the global food supply. This practice is gene editing, not genetically modifying, so it does not yield the same controversy as GMOs. Yi Li is professor of plant science at the University of Connecticut.

As you read, consider the following questions:

1. What crop did Huanglongbing (HLF) devastate with regards to the author's groundbreaking technique?
2. What is gibberellin and what does it affect in plants?
3. Why are annual crops better candidates for the CRISPR technology?

"These CRISPR-Modified Crops Don't Count as GMOs," by Yi Li, The Conversation, May 22, 2018, https://theconversation.com/these-crispr-modified-crops-dont-count-as-gmos-96002.

To feed the burgeoning human population, it is vital that the world figures out ways to boost food production.

Increasing crop yields through conventional plant breeding is inefficient—the outcomes are unpredictable and it can take years to decades to create a new strain. On the other hand, powerful genetically modified plant technologies can quickly yield new plant varieties, but their adoption has been controversial. Many consumers and countries have rejected GMO foods even though extensive studies have proved they are safe to consume.

But now a new genome editing technology known as CRISPR may offer a good alternative.

I'm a plant geneticist and one of my top priorities is developing tools to engineer woody plants such as citrus trees that can resist the greening disease, Huanglongbing (HLB), which has devastated these trees around the world. First detected in Florida in 2005, the disease has decimated the state's US$9 billion citrus crop, leading to a 75 percent decline in its orange production in 2017. Because citrus trees take five to 10 years before they produce fruits, our new technique—which has been nominated by many editors-in-chief as one of the groundbreaking approaches of 2017 that has the potential to change the world—may accelerate the development of non-GMO citrus trees that are HLB-resistant.

Genetically Modified vs. Gene Edited

You may wonder why the plants we create with our new DNA editing technique are not considered GMO? It's a good question.

Genetically modified refers to plants and animals that have been altered in a way that wouldn't have arisen naturally through evolution. A very obvious example of this involves transferring a gene from one species to another to endow the organism with a new trait—like pest resistance or drought tolerance.

But in our work, we are not cutting and pasting genes from animals or bacteria into plants. We are using genome editing technologies to introduce new plant traits by directly rewriting the plants' genetic code.

This is faster and more precise than conventional breeding, is less controversial than GMO techniques, and can shave years or even decades off the time it takes to develop new crop varieties for farmers.

There is also another incentive to opt for using gene editing to create designer crops. On March 28, 2018, U.S. Secretary of Agriculture Sonny Perdue announced that the USDA wouldn't regulate new plant varieties developed with new technologies like genome editing that would yield plants indistinguishable from those developed through traditional breeding methods. By contrast, a plant that includes a gene or genes from another organism, such as bacteria, is considered a GMO. This is another reason why many researchers and companies prefer using CRISPR in agriculture whenever it is possible.

Changing the Plant Blueprint

The gene editing tool we use is called CRISPR—which stands for "Clustered Regularly Interspaced Short Palindromic Repeats"—and was adapted from the defense systems of bacteria. These bacterial CRISPR systems have been modified so that scientists like myself can edit the DNA of plants, animals, human cells and microorganisms. This technology can be used in many ways, including to correct genetic errors in humans that cause diseases, to engineer animals bred for disease research, and to create novel genetic variations that can accelerate crop improvement.

To use CRISPR to introduce a useful trait into a crop plant, we need to know the genes that control a particular trait. For instance, previous studies have revealed that a natural plant hormone called gibberellin is essential for plant height. The GA20-ox gene controls the quantity of gibberellin produced in plants. To create a breed of "low mowing frequency" lawn grass, for example, we are editing the DNA—changing the sequence of the DNA that makes up gene—of this plant to reduce the output of the GA20-ox gene in the selected turf grass. With lower gibberellin, the grass won't grow as high and won't need to be mowed as often.

The CRISPR system was derived from bacteria. It is made up of two parts: Cas9, a little protein that snips DNA, and an RNA molecule that serves as the template for encoding the new trait in the plant's DNA.

To use CRISPR in plants, the standard approach is to insert the CRISPR genes that encode the CRISPR-Cas9 "editing machines" into the plant cell's DNA. When the CRISPR-Cas9 gene is active, it will locate and rewrite the relevant section of the plant genome, creating the new trait.

But this is a catch-22. Because to perform DNA editing with CRISPR/Cas9 you first have to genetically alter the plant with foreign CRISPR genes—this would make it a GMO.

A New Strategy for Non-GMO Crops

For annual crop plants like corn, rice and tomato that complete their life cycles from germination to the production of seeds within one year, the CRISPR genes can be easily eliminated from the edited plants. That's because some seeds these plants produce do not carry CRISPR genes, just the new traits.

But this problem is much trickier for perennial crop plants that require up to 10 years to reach the stage of flower and seed production. It would take too long to wait for seeds that were free of CRISPR genes.

My team at the University of Connecticut and my collaborators at Nanjing Agricultural University, Jiangsu Academy of Agricultural Sciences, University of Florida, Hunan Agricultural University and University of California-San Diego have recently developed a convenient, new technique to use CRISPR to reliably create desirable traits in crop plants without introducing any foreign bacterial genes.

We first engineered a naturally occurring soil microbe, Agrobacterium, with the CRIPSR genes. Then we take young leaf or shoot material from plants and mix them in petri dishes with the bacteria and allow them to incubate together for a couple of days. This gives the bacteria time to infect the cells and deliver the gene editing machinery, which then alters the plant's genetic code.

In some Agrobacterium infected cells, the Agrobacterium basically serves as a Trojan horse, bringing all the editing tools into the cell, rather than engineering plants to have their own editing machinery. Because the bacterial genes or CRISPR genes do not become part of the plant's genome in these cells—and just do the work of gene editing—any plants derived from these cells are not considered a GMO.

After a couple of days, we can cultivate plants from the edited plant cells. Then it take several weeks or months to grow an edited plant that could be planted on a farm. The hard part is figuring out which plants are successfully modified. But we have a solution to this problem too and have developed a method that takes only two weeks to identify the edited plants.

Genetically Designed Lawns

One significant difference between editing plants versus human cells is that we are not as concerned about editing typos. In humans, such errors could cause disease, but off-target mutations in plants are not a serious concern. A number of published studies reported low to negligible off-target activity observed in plants when compared to animal systems.

Also, before distributing any plants to farmers for planting in their field, the edited plants will be carefully evaluated for obvious defects in growth and development or their responses to drought, extreme temperatures, disease and insect attacks. Further, DNA sequencing of edited plants once they have been developed can easily identify any significant undesirable off-target mutations.

In addition to citrus, our technology should be applicable in most perennial crop plants such as apple, sugarcane, grape, pear, banana, poplar, pine, eucalyptus and some annual crop plants such as strawberry, potato and sweet potato that are propagated without using seeds.

We also see a role for genome editing technologies in many other plants used in the agricultural, horticultural and forestry industries. For example, we are creating lawn grass varieties that require less fertilizer and water. I bet you would like that too.

Viewpoint 5

> *"Whilst we may think that sentience is preferable to non-sentience, creating sentient beings with the knowledge that their sentience will largely consist of suffering is cruel."*

We Should Genetically Disenhance Animals Used in Factory Farms

Jonathan Latimer

Genetically altering food may not just mean changing a crop. It might mean changing an animal. And the reasons for that change may not be what you might think. In the following viewpoint, Jonathan Latimer argues that altering animals in factory farms so that they cannot feel pain is an ethical act. This essay was the winner of the University of Oxford's Uehiro Prize for Practical Ethics. When he wrote this essay, Jonathan Latimer was a student at Oxford University.

As you read, consider the following questions:

1. What is disenhancement?
2. What are the primary objections to disenhancement according to the viewpoint?
3. What assumption does the author make before stating his argument?

"Why We Should Genetically 'Disenhance' Animals Used in Factory Farms," by Jonathan Latimer, United Poultry Concerns, March 7, 2018. Reprinted by permission.

I will defend the process of genetic "disenhancement" of animals used for factory farming. I suggest that disenhancement will significantly increase the quality of life for animals in factory farms, and that this benefit is robust against objections that disenhancement is harmful to animals and that it fails to address the immorality of factory farming. Contra to a previous submission, I hope to recast disenhancement as something that ought to be seriously considered on behalf of animals in factory farms.

Currently, the factory farming of livestock animals for human consumption causes a great amount of suffering in those animals. It is widely acknowledged that the conditions many animals face in factory farms are abhorrent. Furthermore, demand for factory-farmed meat is increasing worldwide as developing economies grow more affluent. This will lead to more animals suffering in factory farms in the future. One potential solution to this problem is the "disenhancement" of livestock animals. Disenhancement is a genetic modification that removes an animal's capacity to feel pain. Scientists hope to be able to do this without inflicting any pain at all. So, disenhancement promises to reduce suffering in factory-farmed animals by removing their capacity to feel pain caused by their terrible environment.

However, this solution is not favoured by all. Objections to disenhancement claim that this process is bad for animals and forms part of a morally objectionable institution. These claims are supported by the following arguments:

1. Disability is intrinsically bad; disenhancement causes disability for animals; therefore disenhancement is bad.
2. Factory farming is an immoral process independently of the pain it causes; disenhancement does not change the process of factory farming; therefore disenhancement is not a solution to the immorality of factory farming.
3. Furthermore, disenhancing animals may support or benefit the factory farming industry economically. We should be encouraging the decline of factory farming; therefore we should not disenhance factory farm animals.

For this essay, I am going to assume that factory farming is highly likely to continue in the short term future. As such, my discussion will focus on animals currently in factory farms and those likely to be born into them in the future. This may give the impression that I approve of factory-farming disenhanced animals as a long term goal or the best possible outcome, but I reject this, as I will discuss later on.

Argument 1 claims that disability is intrinsically bad, which seems prima facie intuitive. For example, we live in a society that legally discriminates between disabled and non-disabled people, and provides extra benefits to disabled people in recognition of their status. Whilst this disjunctive conception of disability is useful for societal institutions, it isn't always appropriate to consider specific disabilities as intrinsic harms across all contexts. For instance, we consider a lack of eyesight to be a disability. But this consideration is contingent on actual circumstances; if the human eye had evolved to cause intolerable pain upon contact with light, then we would not consider blindness a disability, but perhaps a benefit. As such, it does not follow that someone has necessarily been harmed by their having what we would typically call a disability, so specific disabilities are not intrinsic harms. We must consider disabilities always within their circumstances, which in this case is a factory farm. In this context, inability to feel pain may be very good for animals, and it shouldn't be considered an intrinsic harm because we would otherwise call it a disability. This line of argument runs parallel to claims that disability should be understood as a mismatch between organism and environment, rather than an inherent defect with the organism.

Another argument as to why disability is intrinsically bad is that disability limits the capacities of the animal, and it is always preferable to have capabilities than to not have them. In the case of disenhancement, the limitation is of the animal's ability to perceive its environment via tactile sensations. We might think that access to diverse channels of perception is a prima facie good thing, it affords variety to experience and endows one with more options of how to pay attention to the world. But in factory farms, where animals are constrained in pens, the animal has little control over the input of experience. The utility of possessing greater varieties of perception is wasted when the external environment is little changing and also pain inducing. Many animals are kept in battery cages for most of their lives, and experience significant pain from being cramped in the same space for too long. Disenhancement would remove this pain, allowing at least for idleness without physical suffering. In the wild, pain has the function of discouraging dangerous behaviour by causing intolerable sensations for brief periods of time. In the unchanging and predator-less environment of the factory farm, this function is useless and merely adds to suffering. The ability of tactile sensation enables the varieties of experience that are doubtlessly the least desirable in the life of a factory farm animal. It would on balance improve the life of the animal if it's very worst experiences were removed, especially given the prevalence of such painful experience, even if doing so limited the capacity of the animal to perceive the environment in certain ways.

Unintuitive consequences do not follow from ceasing to view disability as intrinsic harm, despite the upshot of certain thought-experiments. For instance, if a couple screened their embryos and selected only those with disabilities for no necessary reason, we would be justified in thinking that they had committed a serious wrong. Similarly for disenhancement, because it is an unnecessary disability, it is wrong to create disenhanced animals when there is no need. Although intuitive to an extent, this analogy overlooks important considerations about circumstances. It would be wrong for parents to unnecessarily choose an embryo prone to disability because society remains especially difficult for disabled people. However, it is only wrong insofar as this remains the case. If society changed such that having a certain disability did not lead to harm, causing that disability would not be intrinsically bad. Because it is difficult to imagine how society might be different in such a way, it is easy to conclude that it would always be wrong to cause a disability. But factory farms present the opposite scenario, where the environment is such that disenhancement actually provides a significant benefit. Disenhancement should therefore be seriously considered. It might be responded that disenhancement is never acceptable because experiencing pain prevents you from harming yourself, so depriving factory farm animals of the ability to feel pain will result in more self-injuries. I will address this in my response to Argument 2.

Argument 2 states that even if disenhancement reduces suffering, it does not make factory-farming moral, so we still should not practise factory farming with disenhanced animals. To show that factory farming is bad independently of its causing pain to animals, a previous submission suggests that people with Congenital Insensitivity to Pain with Anhidrosis (CIPA), despite being unable to feel pain, are still harmed by the injuries they incur frequently in daily life. For example, people with CIPA can accidentally bite off their own tongues or fail to notice if they have burned themselves. It is claimed that even though these injuries cause no pain, it is still bad that they happen to people with CIPA —we rightly feel bad for them maiming themselves. Similarly, we are justified in feeling bad for grossly mistreated animals even in the absence of pain.

Whilst I think it is right to point out the seeming inherent inhumanity of factory farm processes, the analogy between this and the injuries of those with CIPA is not consistent. We feel that people with CIPA suffer despite a lack of pain because we recognise that their injuries may still be life-threatening and that society can stigmatise bodily disfigurements. However, the highly restricted environment of a factory farm means that animals face less danger of significantly harming themselves than people with CIPA, and such animals are not subject to stigma. Even with the ability to feel pain, factory farm animals consistently injure themselves as a result of their inhospitable and dangerous living conditions. Factory farming with disenhancement is still deeply unsettling, but our intuitions about the inherent badness of bodily harm are misguided in a context where pain is a near constant feature of conscious experience and has little practical use. Disenhancement does not make factory farming morally sound, but its insufficiency in this regard is not a reason to avoid changing the system to eliminate pointless suffering in the short term.

Building on the claim of Argument 2 that factory farming is inherently immoral, Argument 3 suggests that the implementation of disenhancement would shield factory farming from criticism and strengthen its economic position, leading to the prolonging of an undesirable system. In opting for disenhancement we also tacitly endorse the institution of factory farming and the farmers and scientists who choose to uphold it. Instead, we should explicitly reject all forms of factory farming and push for alternatives.

This argument correctly sheds light on the exploitative and selfish motivations of factory farm owners and scientists in their employment, and it is unfortunate that disenhancement would reduce suffering but also may be in the interest of an exploitative system. However, this unfortunate aspect is no imperative against disenhancement. In reckoning with this issue, the unlikelihood of factory farm practises changing in the near future must be recognised. Vast amounts of people in developing countries are coming to be able to afford meat for the first time, and many will believe that it is their right to demand factory farm products just as those in the developed world have done for decades. In the developed world, vegetarians make up small proportions of total consumers, and cheap factory farmed products are appealing to many people who have to get by on lower incomes. Even if disenhancement leads to reduced moral criticism of factory farming, it is highly likely that demand will remain buoyant. In advocating for the disenhancement of factory farm animals, we recognise that factory farming is likely to continue, and hope that our arguments persuade those people who are determined to produce and consume factory farm products. In the meantime, we can voice opposition to factory farming practises in general and search for alternatives. We don't need to conduct this search whilst animals suffer.

I have responded to the 3 arguments set out at the beginning as to why someone concerned for animal welfare should not accept disenhancement. Specific disabilities should not be considered as intrinsic harms, as the harm caused by a disability often results from the organism's relation to the environment—which is contingent. The processes of factory farming are not made acceptable in and of themselves by disenhancement, but unnecessary suffering is reduced, and we can oppose these processes and work towards their replacement whilst insisting that farmers and scientists immediately reduce suffering with disenhancement.

With the negative case against disenhancement addressed, it can be emphasised that current animals are not harmed by the disenhancement of future animals, and future animals will endure less unnecessary pain. Whilst we may think that sentience is preferable to non-sentience, creating sentient beings with the knowledge that their sentience will largely consist of suffering is cruel. Disenhancement prevents us from creating sentient beings only to exploit them for our own needs, and it also does not stop us from creating sentient beings when they are able to have worthwhile lives, as pets or for conservation. People with concern for animal welfare can make a positive case that disenhancement alleviates the suffering of animals cruelly brought into an existence that guarantees significant pain, and that this does not contradict efforts to replace the system that generates this suffering.

Periodical and Internet Sources Bibliography

The following articles have been selected to supplement the diverse views presented in this chapter.

Jon Cohen, "To Feed Its 1.4 Billion, China Bets Big on Genome Editing of Crops," *Science*, July 29, 2019, https://www.science.org/content/article/feed-its-14-billion-china-bets-big-genome-editing-crops.

Edward Hale, "The Newest Label Coming to a Grocery Store Near You," *The Regulatory Review*, August 20, 2020, https://www.theregreview.org/2020/08/20/hale-newest-label-grocery-store/.

Fiona Harvey, "Genetically Modified Food a Step Closer in England as Laws Relaxed," *The Guardian*, September 29, 2021, https://www.theguardian.com/environment/2021/sep/29/genetically-modified-food-a-step-closer-in-england-as-laws-relaxed.

Greg Jaffe, "What You Need to Know About Genetically Engineered Food," *The Atlantic*, February 7, 2013, https://www.theatlantic.com/health/archive/2013/02/what-you-need-to-know-about-genetically-engineered-food/272931/.

Michael Le Page, "Tomato Is First CRISPR-Edited Food to Go on Sale in the World," *New Scientist*, September 24, 2021, https://www.newscientist.com/article/2291194-tomato-is-first-crispr-edited-food-to-go-on-sale-in-the-world/.

Megan Molteni, "CRISPR Can Help Solve Our Looming Food Crisis: Here's How," *Wired*, August 8, 2019, https://www.wired.com/story/gene-editing-food-climate-change/.

National Geographic Society, "Are Genetically Modified Crops the Answer to World Hunger?" NGS Resource Library, January 28, 2020, https://www.nationalgeographic.org/article/are-genetically-modified-crops-answer-world-hunger/.

Alice Oven, "Is Using Science to Help Animals Adapt to Life on Factory Farms Ever the Solution?" Sentient Media, December 12, 2018, https://sentientmedia.org/changing-animals/.

Nicola Patron and Catherine Price, "Should We Genetically Edit the Food We Eat? We Asked Two Experts," The Conversation, August 11, 2021, https://theconversation.com/should-we-genetically-edit-the-food-we-eat-we-asked-two-experts-162959.

Adam Shriver, "Not Grass-Fed, but at Least Pain-Free," *New York Times*, February 18, 2010, https://www.nytimes.com/2010/02/19/opinion/19shriver.html.

Jay Sullivan, "The Future of Eating: How Genetically Modified Food Will Withstand Climate Change," Natural History Museum, April 22, 2021, https://www.nhm.ac.uk/discover/the-future-of-eating-gm-crops.html.

Mona Zahir, "Pain, Animal Research, and Genetic (Dis) Enchancement," Faunalytics, August 12, 2019, https://faunalytics.org/pain-animal-research-and-genetic-disenhancement/.

For Further Discussion

Chapter 1

1. What are some of the risks posed by allowing parents to edit their children's genes to make them more intelligent, artistic, or athletic, for example? What are the advantages?
2. In the Pew survey discussed in this chapter, religious people were less likely to support the idea of genetic editing of unborn children, even when it was for medical reasons. Why do you think religious people tend to feel this way?
3. How do you imagine a public debate surrounding gene therapy going in the United States? Canada? Other countries? Do you see any reason for international laws to regulate this technology? If so, do you think they would be effective? Why or why not?

Chapter 2

1. Do you think the use of gene-modified animals in medical research has changed the discussion of animals rights? If so, how?
2. China has jumped ahead of the rest of the world in its use of CRISPR, creating human-animal hybrids and even modifying germ lines in a human child. How do you think other nations should respond?
3. Gene editing has been used, among other things, to create a mosquito that could not breed. Most Americans support that use of the technology. Do you? Why or why not? Does knowing that almost half a million people—most of them children—die each year from malaria affect your answer?

Chapter 3

1. One of the motives of scientists working to bring back extinct species, such as the woolly mammoth, is to help restore damaged ecosystems. How might climate change complicate that plan?
2. Some of the people involved in de-extinction programs argue that because humans are responsible for many, if not most, extinctions, we have a moral responsibility to bring these creatures back. Do you agree? Why or why not?
3. Many critics of de-extinction argue that the time and money spent on bringing back extinct species would be better spent trying to save currently endangered species. Can you think of reasons that de-extinction programs might benefit endangered species? What harm might it do?

Chapter 4

1. Proponents of GMO foods claim that this is the only way to be sure we can feed a burgeoning world population. Do you agree? If not, how do you think we should address the problem of world hunger?
2. Of the gene-altering techniques described in this chapter, which do you think is the most promising without introducing the greatest risk?
3. Do you think that making animals unable to feel pain is an appropriate response to the conditions in factory farms? If not, what other solutions do you suggest?

Organizations to Contact

The editors have compiled the following list of organizations concerned with the issues debated in this book. The descriptions are derived from materials provided by the organizations. All have publications or information available for interested readers. The list was compiled on the date of publication of the present volume; the information provided here may change. Be aware that many organizations take several weeks or longer to respond to inquiries, so allow as much time as possible.

The American Society of Human Genetics

3120 Executive Boulevard, Suite 500
Rockville MD 20852
(301) 634-7300
email: society@ashg.org
website: www.ashg.org

The ASHG is an organization working to advance the science of human genetics through research, education, and advocacy.

American Society for Reproductive Medicine

J. Benjamin Younger Office of Public Affairs
726 7th Street SE
Washington, DC 20003
(202) 863-4985
email: Asrm@asrm.org
website: www.reproductivefacts.org

The ASRM is a society for physicians and other professionals in the field of reproductive medicine. It is dedicated to evidence-based education and support of innovative research in keeping with the highest ethical standards.

Biodiversity International

Via dei Tre Denari, 472/a
00054 Maccarese (Fiumicino), Italy
(39-06) 61181
email: biodiversity@cgiar.org
website: www.bioversityinternational.org

Biodiversity International delivers scientific evidence, management practices, and policy options to safeguard agricultural and tree biodiversity to attain sustainable global food and nutrition security.

Canadian Association of Genetic Counsellors

PO Box 52083
Oakville, ON L6L 7N5
Canada
(905) 847-1363
email: cagcoffice@cagc-accg.ca
website: www.cagc-accg.co

The CAGC is a professional organization for genetic counselors, promoting professionalism and public awareness of the profession of genetic counseling.

Cruelty Free International

16a Crane Grove
London
N7 8NN
United Kingdom
email: info@crueltyfreeinternational.org
website: crueltyfreeinternational.org
Cruelty Free International is a UK-based organization that works to end experimentation on animals by exposing the cruelty animals undergo in research labs.

Friends of the Earth

1101 15th Street NW, 11th Floor
Washington, DC 20005
(202) 783-7400
website: www.foe.org

Friends of the Earth is a nonprofit environmental group working for changes that will lead to a healthier and more just world. Recently, the organization joined with other environmental groups to demand tighter regulation of extreme genetic engineering.

Genetic Literacy Project

8 West 126th Street
Suite 3B119
New York, NY 10027
(410) 941-9374
email: info@geneticliteracyproject.org
website: www.geneticliteracyproject.org

The Genetic Literacy Project, a part of the Science Literacy Project, explores the intersection of DNA research and real world applications of genetics with the media and policy worlds in order to disentangle science from ideology. The commitment of the GLP is to promote public awareness and constructive discussion of genetics, biotechnology, evolution, and science literacy.

The Non GMO Project

Contact via website form
(360) 255-7704
website: www.nongmoproject.org

The Non GMO Project is a nonprofit organization committed to building and protecting the food supply primarily through consumer education and outreach.

Revive & Restore

1505 Bridgeway, Suite 203
Sausalito, CA 94965
(415) 289-1000
email: info@reviverestore.org
website: www.reviverestore.org

Revive & Restore is a wildlife conservation organization that works to incorporate biotechnologies into conservation efforts. It is working to restore lost species such as the woolly mammoth and the passenger pigeon.

Wildlife Conservation Society

2300 Southern Boulevard
Bronx, NY 10460
(718) 220-5100
email: membership@wcs.org
website: www.wcs.org

The Wildlife Conservation Society is an international conservation organization that has the goal of preserving the world's largest wild spaces, home to 50 percent of Earth's biodiversity.

Bibliography of Books

Nessa Carey. *Hacking the Code of Life: How Gene Editing Will Rewrite Our Future*. London, UK: Icon, 2019.

Jennifer Doudna and Samuel H. Sternberg. *A Crack in Creation: Gene Editing and the Unthinkable Power to Control Evolution*. Boston, MA: Houghton Mifflin Harcourt, 2017.

Henry T. Greely. *CRISPR People: The Science and Ethics of Editing Humans*. Cambridge, MA: MIT Press, 2021.

Walter Isaacson. *The Code Breaker: Jennifer Doudna, Gene Editing, and the Future of the Human Race*. New York, NY: Simon and Schuster, 2021.

Jim Kozubek. *Modern Prometheus: Editing the Human Genome with CRISPR-Cas9*. Cambridge, UK: Cambridge University Press, 2018.

Sheldon Krimsky. *GMOs Decoded: A Skeptic's View of GMO Foods*. Cambridge, MA: MIT Press, 2019.

Amanda Little. *The Fate of Food: What We'll Eat in a Bigger, Hotter, Smarter World*. New York, NY: Harmony, 2019.

Jamie Metzl. *Hacking Darwin: Genetic Engineering and the Future of Humanity*. Naperville, IL: Sourcebooks, 2019.

Siddhartha Mukherjee. *The Gene: An Intimate History*. New York, NY: Scribner, 2016.

David Quammen. *The Tangled Tree: A Radical New History of Life*. New York: NY: Simon and Schuster, 2018.

Robert D. Saik. *Food 5.0: How We Feed the Future*. Austin, TX: Lioncrest, 2019.

Beth Shapiro. *How to Clone a Mammoth: The Science of De-Extinction*. Princeton, NJ: Princeton University Press, 2021.

Beth Shapiro. *Life as We Made It: How 50,000 Years of Human Innovation Refined—and Redefined—Nature*. New York, NY: Basic Books, 2021.

Jonathan Slack. *Genes: A Very Short Introduction*. Oxford, UK: Oxford University Press, 2014.

James D. Watson. *The Double Helix: A Personal Account of the Discovery of the Structure of DNA*. New York, NY: Simon and Schuster, First Touchstone Edition, 2001.

Carl Zimmer. *She Has Her Mother's Laugh: The Powers, Perversions, and Potential of Heredity*. New York, NY: Penguin, 2018.

Index

A

Ahooja, Raghav, 31–35
alfalfa, GMO, 135
animals, genetic modification of, 53–61, 62–66, 67–73, 74–80, 81–85
Animals (Scientific Procedures) Act (UK), 85
Animal Welfare Act (UK), 85
apples, GMO, 133, 135, 153
AquaBounty Technologies, 138–142
AquAdvantage Salmon, 136, 138–142
Archer, Michael, 97, 102
Aspa Therapeutics, 30

B

Bateman-House, Alison, 25, 27, 29
biodiversity, genetic engineering and, 89–94
Brand, Steward, 108

C

canola, GMO, 133, 135, 146
Cellectis, 144, 146
Church, George, 60, 99, 100, 101, 105
Cibus, 146
Clark, Matt, 115, 116–117
Cohen, Jon, 53–61
Conley, Dave, 141
corn, GMO, 133–134, 145, 152
Cotter, Janet, 77
cotton, GMO, 133, 134, 137, 145
Cowan, Peter, 60
CRISPR-Cas9
  dangers of, 15–16, 52
  explanation of, 15, 63, 124, 151–152
  as potential weapon, 15
CRISPR Therapeutics, 26
Cruelty Free International, 62–66
CTX001 treatment, 26–27

D

Darwin, Charles, 14
David, Eric, 30
de-extinction, 72, 88, 89, 95–106, 107–113
Delborne, Jason, 90–94
Deng Shaoping, 59
Devlin, Robert H., 139
disenhancement, 155–161
DNA, discovery of, 14–15
dodos, 88, 103, 115
Doudna, Jennifer, 56
Draxler, Breanna, 98–99

E

ectogenesis, 34
Effiong, Utibe, 143–148

Esvelt, Kevin, 123, 126, 127
evolution by natural selection, 14, 98
extinct species, bringing back, 72, 88, 89, 95–106, 107–113

F

Federal Food, Drug and Cosmetic Act, 85
Fitch, Chris, 95–106
Fleischer, Robert, 119
Florida panthers, 117–118
Food and Agriculture Organization, 140, 145
foods, genetically modified, 131, 132–137
Friends of the Earth, 76–77, 142
Funk, Cary, 36–43, 67–73
Funk, Chris, 120–121

G

gene drives, 90–94, 122–127
gene therapy trails/"pay-to-play" trials, 24–30
Genetic Biocontrol of Invasive Rodents, 92
genetic diseases, curing of, 15, 18, 21, 25–30, 46
genetic rescue, 114–121
germline altering in humans, 15–16, 19–23, 31–35, 36–43, 44–48
golden rice, 146–147
Great Passenger Pigeon Comeback, 96–97
great prairie chickens, 118

H

Haridy, Rich, 26–27
Hasson, Katie, 48
Heath Hen Project, 101
Hefferon, Meg, 36–43, 67–73
He Jiankui, 55
Hennebold, Jon, 55, 56

I

inbreeding depression, 116, 117, 118
International Commission on the Clinical Use of Human Germline Genome Editing, 44, 45
International Rice Research Institute, 146
International Summit on Human Gene Editing, 20
invasive species, 90, 91–92, 103, 111, 122–127, 140

J

Ji Weizhi, 54, 56

K

Kossel, Albrecht, 14
Kowalski, Kathiann, 122–127
Kuiken, Todd, 127

L

Lai Liangxue, 57, 58, 59, 60, 61
Landsman, Gary, 25, 30
Landsman, Jennie, 29–30
Latimer, Jonathan, 155–161

Lawson, John, 96
Leiden, Jeffrey, 27
Leone, Paola, 28, 29
Li, Yi, 149–154
Lifton, Richard, 47
Logos Environmental, 76, 77

M

Miescher, Johann Friedrich, 14
Moore, Andrew, 89–94
mosaicism, 20
mosquitoes, genetic modification of, 15, 52, 68, 69, 70–71, 125

N

National Human Genome Research Institute, 19–23
Niu Yuyu, 54, 55, 56
Noor, Ramadhani, 143–148
northern white rhinos, 120
Novak, Ben, 96, 97, 101, 102, 103, 106

O

off-target effects, 20, 45, 63, 146
Open Treatments, 28
Orwig, Kyle, 48
outbreeding depression, 117, 118

P

papaya, GMO, 133, 134
passenger pigeons, 96–97, 100–101, 102, 103, 106, 108, 109, 110, 111, 112, 115
Perdue, Sonny, 151
Perls, Dana, 77, 142
Pew Research Center surveys on genetic editing/engineering, 37–43, 67–73
Pimm, Stuart, 117, 118, 120
pink pigeons, 115, 116
Planned Parenthood v. Casey, 34
Poppick, Laura, 114–121
potatoes, GMO, 133, 134, 144–145, 146, 153
Prather, Randall, 57, 58, 59

R

Rack, Jessie, 138–142
Ramesh, Sanath Kumar, 28
Ramsay, Michèle, 46–47
Regalado, Antonio, 24–30
Revive & Restore, 98, 101, 105
Rockwell, Meagan, 29, 30
Roe v. Wade, 32
Ryan, Camilla, 115, 116
Ryder, Oliver, 119–120

S

Saey, Tina Hesman, 44–48, 123
selective breeding, 52, 77, 80, 83, 91
Shapiro, Beth, 100, 101, 103, 104, 105, 108, 109
soybeans, GMO, 133, 134, 146
Strayer, David L., 107–113
sugar beets, GMO, 133, 135
summer squash, GMO, 133, 135
Sundström, Fredrik, 140, 141, 142

Swedish adders, 118
Sygenta, 147

T

TALEN-mediated genome engineering, 145
Third International Conference on Global Warming and Food Security, 144
thylacine/Tasmanian tiger, 97–98, 102

U

US Department of Agriculture, 133, 147
US Food and Drug Administration, 29, 59, 61, 76, 85, 132–137, 138, 139, 141, 142

V

Vazquez, Irina, 140–141
Vertex, 26, 27

W

Wang, Haoyi, 46, 48, 58
Whiteley, Andrew, 118–119
Wilkinson, Anna, 74–80
Wilson, Alexander, 96
Woolly Mammoth Revival, 99
woolly mammoths, 88, 99, 101, 102, 103–105, 108, 110
World Food Program, 144

X

xenotransplantation, 57, 59–61, 71

Y

Yang Hui, 55, 56
Yang Luhan, 60
YourGenome, 81–85

Z

Zhao Jianguo, 58, 60
Zhou Qi, 58